The Unfettered Urologist

The Unfettered Urologist: Endorsements

"Part memoir, part instruction manual, and above all education-al, Dr. Boone shares in *The Unfettered Urologist* her insight into common urology problems with the great integrity I›ve witnessed for 35 years. A must read for patients and doctors alike."

—Raju Thomas, M.D., FACS
President, AUA
Professor and Chair of Urology
Tulane University Medical School

"In *The Unfettered Urologist*, Dr. Boone offers quality informa-tion with entertaining stories about common urology problems. With the ever increasing shortage of practicing urologists, it is more important than ever that primary care providers and their patients have accurate information at their fingertips. I've known Dr. Boone since 1986 and admire her as one of the early women in urology."

—J. Christian Winters, M.D., FACS
H. Eustis Reily Professor and Chairman of Urology
LSU School of Medicine

"*The Unfettered Urologist* is a medical memoir filled with reminis-cences, worldly wisdom, and empiric knowledge providing insight into the ever-changing field of urology. Dr. Boone is an incredibly gifted physician and surgeon, and a gifted writer as well!"

—Meera S. Garcia, M.D.
Chief Medical Officer
Advantia Health

"With *The Unfettered Urologist*, Dr. Martha Boone brings back the empathy, humanity and stories of hope for patients often missing in modern medicine. A fantastic resource for patients (and for practitioners as well), I'm so glad she is sharing her expertise and unique viewpoint with all of us through this book!"

—**Dr. Nicole Cozean**
Founder of PelvicSanity Physical Therapy
Author, *The IC Solution*

"Dr. Boone presents medical information in a clear format that is easily accessible by the public. Her advice is tailored for the patient's understanding of diseases and their treatments, with the patient's safety always her primary concern. Though patients are her target audience, I have learned much from this book."

—**Richard E. Barlow, M.D.**

"Dr. Boone has been a trusted urology colleague for nearly 30 years. The skill she brought to her practice she now brings to this part-memoir, part-textbook for patients. As a senior partner in one of the largest urology groups in the nation, one of the biggest problems we face is misinformation. Her common-sense approach will appeal to patients who need a clear path through a confusing, often biased world."

—**Carl C. Capelouto, M.D.**
Georgia Urology

"*The Unfettered Urologist* is a valuable resource for those looking to address the source of common urology issues. Dr. Boone approaches these difficult and sensitive subjects with a wealth of experience, compassion, and a thorough understanding of the complex nature of urologic dysfunction. Her book provides hope and options."

—**Elizabeth Kemper, PT, MPT, WCS, PRPC**

"This book is a unique personal account of a lifetime of experience as a doctor of urology. It represents the humanistic side of the patient-physician interaction and what a very wise person has learned through the travails and successes of her career. Dr. Boone also includes aphorisms and teachings that apply across the domain of the healing arts."

—Roger Dmochowski, M.D., MMHC, FACS

"Having the good fortune of being a colleague of Dr. Boone for many years, I recognize how well *The Unfettered Urologist* embodies the heartfelt approach that she gave to every patient. A must-read, and the next best thing to being her patient."

—Scott Miller, M.D., MBA

"Brilliant storytelling and raucous humor. Dr. Boone's take on urology is an unexpected total reading experience. Masterful and uniquely written with insider information. A published work worthy of every man and woman."

—Tom A. Dutta
Ph.D. Candidate
Canadian Founder and CEO KRE-AT®
#1 International Best-Selling Author
Radio/Film Producer
TEDx Speaker

"*The Unfettered Urologist* combines Dr. Boone's years of experience and her real-world approach to taking care of patients. It's a book full of curbside consults and practical advice. A must for anyone who doesn't have an urologist on speed dial."

—Sujatha Reddy, M.D.

"Dr. Boone's *The Unfettered Urologist* is extraordinary in sharing valuable insider information about common urology problems. Her book will save you and your loved ones lots of heartache, help you understand basic ways to stay healthy, and avoid the easily preventable catastrophes I see daily in the ICU. Confusion about urinary issues is a part of life. Dr. Boone gives you answers in advance."

—Wes Ely, M.D., MPH
Professor, Medicine and Critical Care
Vanderbilt University
Author, *Every Deep-Drawn Breath*

"Dr Boone has taken various topics in the arcane subspecialty of urology and stitched them together in an organized reference using her 35 years of experience, a problem-solving attitude, empathy for patients, and good humor."

—Barbara N. Croft, M.D.

"What an enjoyable, informative read! Part autobiography, part urology handbook, and all educational, *The Unfettered Urologist* gives valuable information about common urology issues, as well as witty insights on life."

—Susan Jones Kalota, M.D.

"Just as Dr. Boone beautifully captured the essence of life as an intern at Charity Hospital in New Orleans in *The Big Free* (I was there), *The Unfettered Urologist* captures the virtues of old-school doctoring together with state-of-the-art urology. This unique work offers her vast wealth of knowledge and personal experience, creating a must-read for urology patients and the doctors who treat them."

—Frank N. Deus, M.D., FACS, MMM
Urologist and Healthcare Administrator

"Urology problems? Stop searching Dr Google or WebMD and check out Dr. Martha Boone's *The Unfettered Urologist*. It is incredibly informative, clear, and a must-read for anyone who urinates. This profoundly helpful resource combines 35 years of experience in urology to answer your most 'burning' questions."

—Vishal Bhalani, M.D.

"I've been a primary care physician for 30 years and wish I had had this book to refer to. It would have made me look like a star and saved my patients time, unnecessary visits to specialists, and money. Dr. Boone provides invaluable guidance that not only helps doctors but enables patients to take better care of themselves! This book will be my 'go to' for common urological issues."

—Frenesa K. Hall, M.D.
Medical Director
Carolina Pain Relief Center

"Packed with years of experience and memorable patient situations, Dr. Boone's *The Unfettered Urologist* is the ultimate teaching tool for both residents and advanced urologists."

—Martha K. Terris, M.D.
Witherington Distinguished Professor and Chair
Medical College of Georgia

"If you are a primary care doctor or a patient with a urologic problem, I highly recommend two books. The first is *The Unfettered Urologist,* and I suggest you read it twice!"

—Neil Baum, M.D.
Professor, Clinical Urology
Tulane Medical School

"Dr. Boone offers an honest and rare look into the daily practice of urology. A career's worth of wisdom and humor are distilled into practical recommendations, vignettes, and checklists for patients and clinicians."

—Catherine R. deVries, M.D.
Professor, University of Utah

"I've known Dr. Boone for almost 30 years of her career. Martha has an exceptional bedside manner and rapport with her patients. This book will help all current and future patients navigate their health."

—Vahan Kassabian, M.D.
Director, Prostate Center and Advanced Therapeutics
Advanced Urology Institute of Georgia

"I worked with Dr. Boone for years to treat patients with kidney stones. Be sure to take advantage of her wealth of medical and practical knowledge. Patients and providers will both find *The Unfettered Urologist* a great help."

—Shaun Conlon, M.D.
Atlanta Nephrology Associates

"In *The Unfettered Urologist*, Dr. Boone uses her many years of experience to manage over a dozen common urologic problems with a no-nonsense approach. It will aid practitioners and patients alike!"

—Ken Sinervo, M.D.
Medical Director
The Center for Endometriosis Care

"*The Unfettered Urologist* is a beautifully woven book, part memoir and part medical resource guide. Author Martha Boone conveys her knowledge and expertise with humor and empathy. Her deep wisdom will guide me in my focus on prevention and wellness. And seeing healthcare from the physician's vantage point will make me a more empathetic and prepared patient."

—Jeanie P Duncan
Author, *Choosing Me: The Journey Home to My True Self*
President, Raven Group

"Like a conductor directing an orchestra, Dr Boone uses her 35 years of experience to combine the elements of urology into a masterpiece of patient management. Clean, concise, and filled with advice that only a master could provide."

—Carla Roberts, M.D., PhD
Founding Partner, Reproductive Surgical Specialists

"The genital / urinary tract system is one of the most important pillars of the body. Dr. Boone is unique in using a whole-body approach to keep the system healthy and functioning. I always admired her for providing the best care. Her book for physicians, providers, and patients is a rare example of "paying it forward." Ultimately, we will see more patients benefit from the wisdom and knowledge of one of the most dedicated urologists I have known."

—Ceana Nezhat, M.D.
Editor, *Endometriosis in Adolescents*

"Kindness. Compassion. Caring. These are the characteristics Martha Boone brought to her pelvic pain patients. In this book, she provides a treasure trove of insights that will help patients understand their condition, work with their caregivers, and select the most effective therapies. We are blessed that after her retirement, she is sharing this hard-earned wisdom."

—Jill H. Osborne, MA
Founder, Interstitial Cystitis Network

"Bladder control problems, urinary infections, and sexual difficulties affect many of us and can cause so much heartache and confusion! Dr. Boone has created a guide to healing that is as accessible as it is accurate. Bravo, Dr. Boone!"

—Jenelle E. Foote, M.D., FACS
Clinical Assistant Professor of Gynecology,
Morehouse School of Medicine
Clinical Assistant Professor of Family Practice, E
mory School of Medicine

The
UNFETTERED
Urologist

WHAT I NEVER HAD TIME TO TELL YOU
IN A FIFTEEN-MINUTE OFFICE VISIT

Martha B. Boone, M.D.

NEW YORK

LONDON • NASHVILLE • MELBOURNE • VANCOUVER

The UNFETTERED Urologist

What I Never Had Time to Tell You in a Fifteen Minute Office Visit

Published in New York, New York, by Morgan James Publishing. Morgan James is a trademark of Morgan James, LLC. www.MorganJamesPublishing.com

This book contains the opinions and ideas of the author. The book intends to give primary care providers, patients, and their families the author's opinions of how our medical system works and what they can do independently before seeking medical advice from a urologist.

The book does not provide medical services. The book is not intended to replace the advice of your medical professional who is familiar with your specific case.

Throughout the book, several companies, health care providers, and products are mentioned. The author has no current financial arrangement with any of these entities.

The author and publisher disclaim all responsibility for any liability or risk incurred by consequence of using any of the content in this book. Any and all advice should be approved by your professional medical advisor.

Proudly distributed by Ingram Publisher Services.

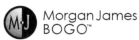

Morgan James BOGO™

A **FREE** ebook edition is available for you or a friend with the purchase of this print book.

CLEARLY SIGN YOUR NAME ABOVE

Instructions to claim your free ebook edition:
1. Visit MorganJamesBOGO.com
2. Sign your name CLEARLY in the space above
3. Complete the form and submit a photo of this entire page
4. You or your friend can download the ebook to your preferred device

ISBN 9781636980720 paperback
ISBN 9781636980737 ebook
Library of Congress Control Number: 2022947814

Cover Design by:
Rachel Lopez
www.r2cdesign.com

Interior Design by:
Chris Treccani
www.3dogcreative.net

Front Cover Photo by:
Karen Burns

Author Photo by:
Jesse Boone

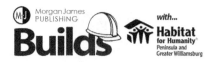

Morgan James PUBLISHING Builds with... **Habitat for Humanity® Peninsula and Greater Williamsburg**

Morgan James is a proud partner of Habitat for Humanity Peninsula and Greater Williamsburg. Partners in building since 2006.

Get involved today! Visit: www.morgan-james-publishing.com/giving-back

Dedication

If you have a great hospital, it's because you have great nurses.

This book is dedicated to the unsung heroes: the amazing nurses and technicians at Charity Hospital in New Orleans, Tulane Medical Center, Ochsner Clinic, University of California-Davis, the Veterans Administration, The Medical College of Georgia, and the nurses in the Northside Hospital network in Atlanta, Alpharetta, and Cumming, who helped me and my patients for my entire career. You know who you are.

I could never have been successful without great nurses assisting me every step of the way.

CONTENTS

"There lives more faith
in honest doubt, believe me,
than in half the creeds."

Chapter I

Never Enough Time

"The two most powerful warriors
are patience and time."

– LEO TOLSTOY

W hy would I quit my job as a very successful surgeon and spend my time writing about what I never had time to tell my patients in the office?

After thirty-five years as a urologist, over nine-thousand surgeries, over one hundred and seventy-five thousand patient visits, and six jobs in four cities, my biggest frustration was not having enough time with my patients. I often left the exam room craving more time to share non-medical and non-science information. I regretted not having adequate time to listen to everything the patient wanted to say. I was disappointed at having only an average of fifteen minutes with each person.

For many years I felt crushed under the burden of ever-increasing regulation from outside entities that left me feeling a sense of emptiness and inadequacy. I always gave my best scientific and medical advice. I stuck strictly with the script of what was known from medical science about a patient's disease. I diligently studied every X-ray and blood test. I carefully examined each part of the body involved in the patient's problem. I kept up with all the latest technology and took regular courses to keep my knowledge up to date.

Year after year I won the TOP DOC contests for my excellent patient care. Yet, I had so much more to give my patients, but no time. It was my duty to make sure they knew the scientific opinion. It was my greatest desire to give them my practical knowledge, my intuition, and my opinion from extensive experience.

Many patients feel great frustration when interfacing with our medical system, but don't realize why. Doctors in America are paid by something called work relative value unit (RVU), which means we are expected to produce a certain amount of work in a short period of time. If we don't produce enough relative value units, we can't pay our office bills. The cost of practicing medicine goes up every year. Every year, the amount of time all medical professionals spend documenting information for the government and insurance payors increases. The time spent documenting is taken away from the time we'd spend listening and talking to the patient. We feel the pressure. The system is not always conducive to assisting in your best health. My own and my patients' frustration grew over the years.

In 2020, I'd been a medical doctor since 1985. I decided to leave my practice to take a yearlong sabbatical in hopes of curing my frustration. I wanted to fulfill one of my lifetime goals—to travel the world while my husband and I were able. I had watched close friends and colleagues suffer unexpected diseases that made their retirement miserable.

One of the reasons I love being a doctor is that I love studying people. I want to see where they live, what they eat, how they work and raise their families. I want to understand their spiritual beliefs. I want to hear as many languages, eat as many different types of food, hear as many types of music, and see as much art as possible. We mapped out a full year of traveling the globe to experience the many varieties of the human condition. One month after we started our sabbatical, Covid-19 hit and our plans evaporated.

Leaving my patients had been bittersweet. I wanted to write a love letter to them. I wanted to thank them for trusting me and being my patient. So I decided that since it was deemed not safe to travel, to write some of the things I always wanted to say, but never had the time.

Please know that I'm not offering medical advice in this book. Every chapter is my opinion. Much of it is not supported by the strictest science. Nothing here should replace sound medical advice from a doctor who knows your particular situation. Nor does anything here represent the opinions of any organization with which I have ever been affiliated. At some junctures, I actually go against the advice of my previous governing agencies.

This book embodies the opinions and practical knowledge of a woman who has devoted forty-four years of her life to science and thirty-five years to medicine. Many have called me a trailblazer for being among the first one hundred women to be board certified in urology. I define myself as a nerdy little bookworm who loves science, loves people, and was blessed enough to find a job allowing me to serve both passions.

I hope to provide information on how to think about illness and help yourself in our medical system, and to offer tools for self-care. There are many means of healing that won't be found in the average doctor's office. If you take nothing else from this book, please do not ignore blood in your urine and DO NOT SMOKE.

I hope you find something in this book to help you, or at least a story to make you laugh or cry.

Chapter II

Three Doctors in One

"Make the most of yourself, for that is all there is of you."
– RALPH WALDO EMERSON

I'm not sure exactly when it happened. But sometime between 1996 and 2010, it became necessary for me to be three varieties of *the doctor*.

For the first eleven years of my practicing medicine, I was one type of doctor: the expert. I was a highly educated professional scientist to whom you brought your medical problems and trusted your deepest secrets. You took my advice, most of the time, and usually got better. The relationship was simple.

And then, everything started to shift. I blame the internet.

Young people without a firm grasp of eighth-grade biology brought inch-thick stacks of paper copied from the internet to their office visits. They argued and told me of their diagnoses as determined by them and Google. If I didn't seem to know every line of what was gleaned from their internet search, I was deemed inadequate and they moved on to the next doctor. As they stomped out of the office refusing to pay their co-pay, they'd walk right past my wall of impressive diplomas without giving them a glance, then sit in their cars and write scathing internet reviews to let the world know of my idiocy.

At first, I found these interactions amusing. Then I was incredulous. Finally, I fought to hide my anger. The under-thirty crowd became a mystery to me. To be their doctor, I had to constantly do battle with their internet searches. Unbeknownst to me, Google was god to them. I was hurt, lost, and confused. How could they trust an unknown entity but distrust a real human, with advanced education they could easily validate, sitting right in front of them?

At the same time, the patients from 30 to 65 years old sought a partner in health care. This was my own age group and I related best to them. They respected my education. They knew I knew more than they did. But it was their body and nobody was going to tell them to do anything that did not sound correct.

This kind of patient wanted a coach or a trusted advisor, like the person who did their finances. Most listened respectfully, asked a mile-long list of questions, and went home to consider my advice and decide what they would or would not do. If we could not come to a mutually agreed-upon course of action, I'd suggest a second opinion and they'd accept that idea. This age group mostly wanted time to discuss everything they had read and have me explain basic science, biology, and medicine to them, so that they could buy into my mostly trusted advice. Nearly all of these patients came back to see me and followed my suggestions. Occasionally, one decided the second opinion doctor was more to their liking, but the interaction was civil, honest, and straightforward.

Again at this same time, I treated the over-65 crowd much as I always had. I loved my older patients best, though they were often irascible or even mean. They'd seen it all and weren't impressed with much. They had survived wars, depressions, and deaths of loved ones, financial gains and losses. They were in the last phase of life, trying to keep their dying bodies going, and had no time for fancy words. They came with a list of complaints and expected solutions.

Usually their primary care physician had discovered something with which they needed help. They respectfully relayed their stories and expected me to respond like a great oracle and tell them what to do. Recognizing the personal nature of the doctor-patient relationship, they wanted me to know about their grandson's baseball expertise as well as their kidney stone attack. This group didn't argue with me, but they expected an answer. They rarely asked for another opinion. If their primary care doctor told them I was the one to solve their problem, they trusted that doctor, if not me. They didn't hop from one doctor to another. But, by God, they expected me to figure things out.

Before I'd fully realized my need to be three doctors in one, I had a few shocks. One day I was performing a vaginal exam on a 22-year-old who clutched her phone as I explained what was going to happen. I don't know when everyone began clutching their phones. But, I was familiar with the behavior. It reminded me of a pediatric patient holding their favorite doll or bear for comfort. People her age held tight to their phones at all times. I thought nothing of it.

When I was sure she was comfortable with the planned pelvic exam, I moved to my rolling stool to position myself between her legs. My nurse made ready the ubiquitous K-Y jelly. I was gloved, sitting at eye level with the entrance to her vagina, and completely focused on discovering the cause of her urethral pain.

I explained what I was doing before I did it and she seemed relaxed about the experience. As I pulled my gloved fingers out of her vagina, her crotch exclaimed, "What did you find, doctor?"

Entranced in my deep focus on the source of her problem, I imagined her vagina was talking to me! I was so startled that I pushed back quickly, jammed my rolling stool against the wall behind me and slammed my head into the wall.

As my head bobbed back into position, the vagina continued to talk as if nothing strange had occurred. When I gained my composure, I realized this young woman had me on facetime with her mother. Her mother had been watching me perform a pelvic exam on her daughter.

I was speechless. I felt disrespected and violated. I was no longer the trusted expert. Without realizing it, I had become a new kind of doctor, and the expectations of me were nothing I understood.

No matter your age, I advise the following to improve your interactions with our medical system and your doctor:

- Come prepared for your visit by reading a trusted medical site. Many doctors have information on their websites about the conditions they treat. Spend time reading that information if it pertains to your problem. There is much information that is incorrect on the web. Avoid any site that is not recommended by a medical professional you know. Lots of folks are masquerading as doctors and many of them have impressive yet incorrect sites.

- Think about why you seek advice and write the questions you want answered.

- Realize your doctor is pressured for time. The better you organize yourself, the better your visit will be. Bring any relevant X-rays, lab results, or notes from other doctors pertaining to your current condition. If you are seeking a second opinion, tell the doctor. No confident doctor should ever be insulted by your desire for a second opinion.

- Take notes. I've been impressed with how little people remember from their visits. I think people are afraid the doctor is going to tell them something life-changing and many can't listen because of fear. Ask for printed material or a website to review what has been suggested.
- If possible, bring someone with you to any visit that is likely to result in life-altering information. Two calm heads are better than one. Ask them to take notes too.
- If your doctor is young and you are older, remember the young doctor has always been in the world of the internet and technology. When they turn their back to you to type in the medical record, it's not a personal affront. Every generation has slightly different social rules. If you are young and your doctor is older, be patient. They might not be as adept at technology as you, but their experience with medicine is very valuable. The visit will go better if you appreciate their experience and are patient with them about their inadequacy with technology.
- Remember the goal of the visit: You are there to seek information. You never have to do what the doctor advises. An open mind is an invaluable tool. Stay as relaxed and receptive as possible to get the most information. Afterwards, you can decide whether to trust them and follow their advice, get another opinion, or consider a nontraditional healing route. Of course, if you are in the throes of a true medical emergency go to the best hospital in town and do what you are told.
- Remember that all healthcare professionals detest having to spend so much time documenting the electronic medical record. But unless you want a concierge doctor and plan to pay all your bills out of your own pocket, it is

a necessary evil. If you have multiple medical problems or wish to budget for the best care, you might find your money well spent with a concierge primary doctor. To my knowledge, there are no concierge urologists.

Chapter III

"Doc, my urine is red!"

*"The art of medicine consists in amusing the patient
while nature cures the disease."*

– VOLTAIRE

I wish I could say medicine has greatly advanced in all areas
since the time of Voltaire and the Enlightenment, but in some
areas, it has not.

This chapter is about hematuria or blood in the urine. Ninety
percent of the people with microscopic blood in the urine have no
serious medical condition. Five percent have a benign, i.e., non-
cancerous cause for the blood, including kidney stones, kidney
cysts, urinary tract infections, and medical or nephrology issues.
But five percent of people with blood in their urine have kidney,
ureter, bladder, urethra, or prostate cancer.

Unfortunately, all the organs of the urinary tract are buried
deep in the body and not easily accessed like the breasts, eyes,
skin, and extremities. So, a physical examination does not give the
doctor much information. Even with deep palpation of the body,
doctors usually cannot feel a kidney cancer.

If you have blood that you can see with your naked eye (gross hematuria), smoked for over five years or inhaled lots of second-hand smoke, or are over forty years of age, the risk of something serious goes up. If you have any of these risk factors and blood in your urine, it's prudent to see a urologist soon.

Patients with blood invisible to the naked eye (but seen in the microscope) and no risk factors are the most difficult group to follow and treat. I've had blood in my urine for twenty years. I have undergone the entire workup for hematuria three times and all tests have been normal. But, in that same timeframe, two close friends who were doctors have died and many have been treated for urinary tract cancers detected only by a microscopic urinalysis.

One morning my phone rang at six a.m. and one of my favorite anesthesiologists was on the line. I'd been expecting a call about a patient I'd scheduled for surgery that day. Instead, a shaky and weak voice said, "Hi, It's me. I'm sorry to bother you so early. But I have blood in my urine and I'm scared to death." He's one of the most skilled and best loved doctors in our system. He's kind and smart and a team player. When I'm in the operating room and he's doing my patient's anesthesia, I know I can relax because he always does a great job. Hearing him worried and frightened brought me to full attention.

I thought he might be a nervous nelly. He'd never smoked, never been around smokers, and was very healthy. I thought there was likely nothing wrong with him but he was my friend and I didn't want him to worry. I said, "Meet me at the office in 30 minutes and I'll take a look."

I warmed up my ultrasound machine while drinking my coffee, thinking we were probably wasting our time. He arrived, we hugged, and I checked his urine. It showed blood, but then I had blood in my urine too. I still wasn't worried; after all, there was a ninety-five percent chance he had nothing seriously wrong.

Even though the recommended test for kidney cancer is a computerized axial tomography (CAT scan) with and without IV contrast, I frequently did ultrasound in my office to get an idea of whether the patient might have a stone or not. My good friend laid his long, lanky body face down on the examining table, and as I applied the warm jelly to his back, I thought I'd at least reassure him before he headed to work.

We joked with each other as we always did. I moved the ultrasound probe around on his back for ten seconds and had to fight back a gasp. I saw a softball-sized mass protruding from his kidney. My hand shook while I stalled for time and moved the probe from one kidney to the other.

After a few minutes, he began to panic. "What? What is it? Martha, you're not talking! What do you see?" asked my dear friend the anesthesiologist.

I've never been one to hide the truth from any patient. I'm also not particularly good at cushioning blows. I don't coddle myself, my family, or my patients. And now my buddy was my patient.

"It looks like a big kidney tumor. We need to get a CAT scan to confirm. I want one of the robotic guys to help us with this," I said.

As I wiped the jelly from his back and helped him pull down his shirt, his eyes were wide and his breathing fast and shallow. His first concern was his wife and his family. I have good reason to love and respect this man.

This story has a happy ending. We caught the cancer in time. One of the best robotic urologic surgeons in the south east took out his kidney and he's fine. I am very grateful we did not ignore the blood in his urine!

Another physician, a gastroenterologist who was my friend for over 20 years, made different choices. When blood was found in his urine, he decided not to be evaluated, thinking, "ninety percent of people with blood in their urine have nothing wrong with them." He played ice hockey, had never smoked or lived with smokers, ate a healthy diet, was never overweight, and assumed the blood in his urine was from contact sports. He was wrong. He was in the five percent. Despite receiving the best care available, he died a preventable death at age 55 from metastatic bladder cancer. His last words on our last phone call were, "I love you and thanks for being my friend." I remember him every time a patient refuses to be evaluated for blood in their urine. His death made the workup of hematuria very personal to me.

HOW DO WE DETERMINE THE CAUSE OF THE BLOOD IN A PATIENT'S URINE?

- Urinalysis – Under the microscope, we look at your urine for blood cells, infection cells, and crystals that could indicate infection or kidney stones. Sometimes the chemical or dipstick test is not accurate. So, it's important to always make a diagnosis of blood in the urine with a microscopic examination.
- Urine culture – Tests for infectious causes of blood.
- Urine cytology – Tests for cancer cells in the urine. Cancer can be missed with this test. That's called a false negative. If this test is positive, you likely do have cancer as the false positive rate for this test is quite low. There are many other urine markers available, but so far none have been able to replace the standard testing suggested here.
- Fluorescence in situ hybridization (FISH) – A test sometimes given smokers with gross hematuria to test for chro-

mosomal abnormalities of their urine cells to look for the propensity to have bladder cancer. Again, if negative it does not guarantee you don't have a urinary tract tumor. But if the test is positive, the likelihood of there being a cancer somewhere in your urinary tract increases.

- Blood testing – Looks for kidney disease, prostate cancer, and risk factors for kidney stone formation. There is currently no blood test able to predict urinary tract tumors.

- Computed Axial Tomography (CT or CAT scan) – X-ray test for kidney, ureter, or bladder cancer, or stones.

- Magnetic resonance imaging (MRI) – Often used if you have an iodine contrast allergy or to better stage a tumor found on an ultrasound or CAT scan. "Staging" means getting more information about the extent of your tumor to determine the best course of action. MRI is very accurate for tumor diagnosis, but does not demonstrate kidney stones as well as CT.

- Cystoscopy – A fiber optic scope is introduced into the urethra to look at the bladder from the inside. If a CT shows a bladder tumor, a cystoscopy may be done in the operating room with anesthesia and be combined with bladder biopsy or tumor removal. If the CT looks normal, cystoscopy is sometimes done in the office with a very small scope. The patient would need both CT and cystoscopy as thirty percent of small bladder tumors can be missed on CT.

MY ADVICE:

- Don't smoke or use tobacco products of any type. The urinary tract filters out liquid wastes and the bladder stores them until it's convenient to release them. We are absolutely certain that the use of tobacco products increase the chance of urinary tumors.

- If you have relatives with kidney or bladder cancer, have your urine checked every year at your physical, because kidney and bladder cancer may carry a genetic association. The genetic association is not as strong as with prostate cancer or breast cancer, but there does seem to be one.
- If you ever see blood in your urine and are not menstruating, see a urologist. Even if you only see the blood one time, it is an ominous finding that should never be ignored.

The tests described above are costly, slightly invasive, and time-consuming. But, I chose to have them three times because I don't want to be the patient who dies from a preventable problem. So, just as I get my workup, I strongly advise my patients to get theirs, even though the tests will be normal much of the time.

Each of us has to decide how we are going to interact with our medical system. Are you going to see your doctor only when you have a problem that's obvious? If you choose that route, you are unlikely to have *unnecessary tests*. But, if you do develop a serious medical problem, it might be caught too late for treatment. Or are you like me and want to be proactive and preventative about health issues? If so, you'll have many *normal* tests, but will be much less likely to die of preventable diseases. I prefer to keep my organs and be as healthy as possible, so I get regular checkups and have the testing that is suggested by my colleagues.

How do doctors decide what to recommend to their patients? For the problem of hematuria, a committee of professionals meets every three to five years and reviews the world's scientific literature on the subject. This group looks in detail at the various available tests, how the diseases are behaving in the population, what tests give the highest yield, and where we are falling short in diagnosis and management. Then, after much deliberation, the committee makes recommendations. Individual doctors are not bound to follow them, but they do provide *best practice guidelines* to assist primary care doctors, gynecologists, and internal medicine doctors.

You might have experienced your doctor making one suggestion about your hematuria one year and a different suggestion the next. This is because doctors undergo continuing medical education (CME) and advise their patients based on the latest available knowledge. Each doctor is allowed to make their best recommendation for their patient relying on detailed information about that person's particular case. If you have blood in your urine, you are very likely to be sent to urology. I advise you to go.

Chapter IV

Interstitial Cystitis, Bladder Pain, and Prostatodynia

Painful Bladder Syndrome/Chronic Prostatitis-Prostate Pain

"Adversity is the first path to truth."

– LORD BYRON

P ain is a fascinating topic, particularly if you're not the person who's suffering.

I've seen thousands of patients with pelvic pain since 1985. Even when I was a resident and knew little, women faculty members, residents' wives and girlfriends, nurses, and female patients sought me out. They believed my being female gave me more compassion and insight into their bladder pain. The average urologist might see ten percent of their patients for bladder or pelvic pain. At times in my practice, thirty percent of my patients had been diagnosed with interstitial cystitis, i.e., pelvic pain syndrome, or chronic prostatitis.

One thing I know for certain is that the experience of pain is an individual response. Many years ago I traveled to Ethiopia to perform vesicovaginal fistula repair surgery for women in the remote city of Wolaita Sodo. The hospital where we worked is eight hours south of the capital of Addis Ababa, and is approximately equidistant to Somalia, Kenya and Djibouti. The trip was on dirt roads that required jeeps to carry extra fuel on their roofs because no services were available in the isolated area. We passed dirt hut after dirt hut during our scorching and dusty 200-mile trek south.

I went to this remote place for my fiftieth birthday to pay back a debt for the amazing education I've had and to challenge my surgical skills in reconstruction to help as many women as possible. Our team raised money for a year to pay the local hospital to allow us to repair vesicovaginal and recto-vaginal fistulas. The continent of Africa, and indeed the world, has many women with urine and feces running down their legs due to unattended birth from the lack of adequate obstetrics care. Many women marry young before their pelvis is fully developed and able to accommodate childbirth. During their attempted childbirth, they labored, sometimes for days, with the baby unable to exit their narrow pelvis. With no experienced nurse midwife or obstetrician available, the obstructed labor tore the bladder tissue and rectal tissue by rubbing them repetitively on the pelvic bones in an effort for the baby to be born. (If you are interested in this topic and want to learn more, watch the documentary *A Walk to Beautiful*).

Many of these unfortunate women were viewed in their communities as cursed by God and were frequently abandoned by their husbands and left to fend for themselves. The more fortunate women died during the process. The baby usually died also.

While the trip was extraordinary in many ways, one of the things I found most remarkable was the patients' response to pain. The women walked miles across hilly areas of sub-Saharan Africa. They came from all over the area and spoke many different dialects while our interpreter spoke only Amharic. We operated on them with communication so poor that they could not have understood what we were going to do. They simply knew we were American-trained surgeons and had come to help them.

The surgeries are invasive and required large abdominal, vaginal, and rectal incisions. In theory and in practice, the surgery should hurt terribly. To my unending shock, when I checked on the patients the next day, I'd find them sitting up in bed with huge incisions, multiple tubes, and a big smile on their face asking for NO pain medication. I was dumbfounded. If a similar procedure had been done in America, the pain team would have been involved for days and the patient would have gone home with strong pain medication.

I learned from my time in Ethiopia that pain is subjective and individual. I wish I could have spoken the languages of the women to better understand their experience. Our only language was that of their big smile and my concerned eyes. In their eyes, I saw trust. Their appreciative family members often dropped to the ground and kissed my feet. Their trust, expectations, and gratitude were greater than I received from many patients back home.

If you want to learn more about this hospital and have any interest in helping, a link to its website is on the resources page of my website. The doctors there have made enormous progress since our time there. Your donations would be appreciated.

This chapter is not about acute pain caused from incisions from recent surgery or injury. Our topic is the more complex topic of chronic pelvic pain. I mentioned our time in Ethiopia to demonstrate that pain is a subjective response that varies from one person to another and from one culture to another. The degree of injury does not always correlate to the individual patient's experience of pain.

CAUSES OF CHRONIC PELVIC PAIN:
- Interstitial cystitis or IC (painful bladder syndrome)
- Endometriosis
- Pelvic floor dysfunction (muscle spasm)
- Prior surgery (scarring and adhesions)
- Pelvic congestion syndrome
- Pelvic inflammatory disease
- Chronic constipation
- Chronic bladder or vaginal infection
- Colitis (irritable bowel syndrome)
- Neuralgia (pain from damage)
- Fibromyalgia (Muscle pain)
- Uterine fibroids
- Prostatitis (infection or inflammation)

My experience with pelvic pain could fill volumes. There were points in my career when I thought the patients were crazy. On particularly frustrating days, I thought I might be crazy. When a problem is hard to diagnose and harder to treat, the patient, their family, and the doctor share a microcosm of frustration. The truth lay in the realization that we were attempting to treat a multifaceted problem with a few inadequate tools.

Here, I seek to summarize as simply as possible what I have learned about this complex problem of pelvic pain. In many patients, I found an inciting event. With some it was a bladder, vaginal, or prostate infection. With others it was a bladder catheter.

With many, there was a history of trauma such as pelvic fracture, broken coccyx, sexual or emotional abuse. Sometimes the inciting event was prior pelvic surgery. Occasionally it was childbirth. Rarely, the patient had no recollection of anything that could have led to their misery.

I witnessed a familiar cycle with my chronic pelvic pain patients. They'd start out hopeful. *If I just find the right doctor, or the right procedure, or the right drug, this pain will go away.* Sometimes, the more we did, the worse they got. Later in the process, the patients were angry and incredulous. *Why can't you fix my problem?* Then, they became desperate and willing to try anything. The desperation gave way to depression. *Is the rest of my life going to be like this?* Marriages crumbled due to painful intercourse and loss of sexuality. Pain made it impossible for the patients to sleep and function. Many could not focus to work or care for their children and home. At times, they felt life was not worth living.

If what we called interstitial cystitis went untreated, the cycle ceased with no medical intervention 15–20% of the time. The symptoms simply disappeared. If chronic pelvic pain was left unchecked, some patients spiraled down into hopelessness.

I was in Italy on vacation one spring when my medical assistant called with the news that, "One of our IC patients faxed a suicide note to our office!" The note described the patient as not being able to cope anymore. She was a beautiful young woman with a lovely husband and three little children.

I spent the day trying to locate her family and sent the police to her home for a wellness check. When she was found, she was dead. Her pelvic pain won and her family was left to deal with the aftermath. I wish I could report that she was the only patient to commit suicide over their pelvic pain. The impact suicide has on the family and even the healthiest, most highly functioning health-care professionals cannot be overstated. The family and the health care team need professional assistance to handle the post-traumatic event emotions.

Despite these terrible losses, we have made much progress. Most urologists and gynecologists don't want to treat chronic pelvic pain. Success is not guaranteed, and when answers are difficult to find, the patients can be a fractious and unruly group. I became known as someone willing to try to help them and *think outside of the box.* Other doctors knew I was willing to try and they sent patients to me in droves. The ones I could help loved me and the ones I could not help hated me. It was a challenge and some days a curse.

If you have chronic urinary frequency, urgency and pelvic or prostate pain, what should you do?

- Avoid eating tomatoes, chocolate, caffeine, bananas, and fruit juices, and consider following an interstitial cystitis elimination diet. Avoid vitamins, particularly vitamin C and turmeric, when you have urinary frequency and urgency.

- Make sure you don't have an infection. Your gynecologist or general doctor will culture your urine. If your cultures are negative, do not take antibiotics because they may make your condition worse. Well-meaning primary care and urgent care doctors want to do something to help you and some will give antibiotics while waiting for the culture to return. Resist repetitive antibiotics when your cultures are negative. Destroying your gut microbiome, getting chronic yeast infections, and getting resistant organisms is the end result of taking antibiotics you don't need.

- If you are a female, get evaluated by a gynecologist who treats endometriosis all the time. Endometriosis is a common cause of pelvic pain and there are excellent doctors to help with this disease. The results are very good in the hands of an expert.

- No matter the cause of your pelvic pain, pelvic floor physical therapy (PT) can help. PT has by far been the most effective treatment for my pelvic pain patients. I'm not trained in physical therapy and can't completely explain how it works. The way I explained the use of PT for pelvic pain to my patients was simplistic but effective: When the body has pain caused by any condition, it reacts with muscle spasm in an attempt to splint the area and reduce the pain. Repetitive muscle spasms cause inflammation in the area, which starts a vicious cycle that worsens the pain problem. By manually relaxing the pelvic muscles and teaching the patient stretching techniques, the cycle can be broken and pain diminished. Be sure you consult a physical therapist with special training in the pelvic floor. Know that if you are female, the visits will require a vaginal and likely a rectal examination for diagnosis. Males may also need a rectal exam.

- Avoid the Kegel exercise program if you have pelvic pain. Kegels are great for preventing urinary incontinence but they often made pain patients' symptoms worse. Your PT will help you determine what types of exercise and stretches are best for you.

- I cannot stress enough the importance of having a good bowel program if you have chronic pelvic pain. An unemptied lower bowel weighs heavy on the pelvic organs. Straining to have a bowel movement induces pelvic muscle spasm. Your physical therapist can help with the mechanics of defecation. If constipation is chronic, see a gastroenterology (GI) specialist to be sure nothing is seriously wrong. They can also help with your bowel program. In my experience, probiotics and good diet solved most mild constipation. Some patients benefited from daily magnesium citrate ingestion at night. Others use fiber supplements. Some needed prescription medication to empty their bowels. If your constipation is not resolved, your pelvic pain is unlikely to fully resolve.

Chronic pain causes *upregulation of your nervous system.* This means that over time, your body reacts with greater intensity to minor stimuli. Your sensitive bladder can normally discern when it is partially full, totally full, and about to leak urine. Your bowel is so sensitive that it differentiates between gas, liquid, and solid stool.

There's a plethora of nerve input coming and going from the pelvis. In chronic pain, the nerves are oversensitive and send messages to the brain that are out of proportion to the stimulus. For example, your bladder might signal your brain it's full when it is not. This faulty information causes you to go to the bathroom every 15 minutes. Once these nerves are firing out of control, how do we turn that around?

TREATMENT OPTIONS FOR AN OVERACTIVE NERVOUS SYSTEM:
- Hypnotherapy
- Acupuncture
- Chiropractic care
- Physical therapy
- Stress reduction techniques
- Psychiatric care and medications
- Meditation
- Guided imagery

- Long, slow periods of mild exercise
- Diet (IC diet, anti-inflammatory diet)

ORAL AGENTS TO HELP SYMPTOMS:
- NSAIDs (Naprosyn, Motrin)
- Over the counter or prescription antihistamines
- Calcium glycerophosphate (Prelief)
- Single dose sodium bicarbonate (1 tsp. of baking soda in 10 oz. of warm water. I suggest you not do this more than once per month as it is a heavy salt load)
- Oral aloe vera. Desert Harvest aloe vera (three pills in the morning and three in the evening) was the most popular aloe product among my patients.
- CystoProtek (chondroitin sulfate, sodium hyaluronate, glucosamine sulfate, quercetin, rutin).

In my experience, each of the above treatments helped patient symptoms of intense frequency, urgency, and pelvic pain, on average 60% of the time. If the patient saw no improvement in frequency, urgency and burning within a month, there was no benefit in continuing the oral products.

I have no experience with medical marijuana or CBD oil and cannot make suggestions regarding these products. It is my belief that these treatments should be low on the list of options to try in cases of recalcitrant symptoms.

What seldom worked in my hands was the most recommended medical treatment in the 1990's, hydro-distension. For the first 10 years I treated painful bladder syndrome, I was terrified I might overlook a small bladder cancer. Due to that fear, I took every patient to the operating room to biopsy the bladder, perform hydrodistension (stretch the bladder), and instill anti-inflammatory agents in the bladder. The procedure reassured me that I had not missed bladder cancer but helped the patient's symptoms only 30% of the time. And, sadly enough, half the patients were temporarily worse! I never discovered an undiagnosed bladder cancer. Even though this surgery was the recommended procedure at the time, I quickly lost enthusiasm for it. It seemed to me (and this idea is not in the medical literature that I searched) that the trauma of the surgery irritated the bladder in many people. For the folks in whom it worked, it was almost miraculous. They'd awaken in the recovery room feeling better.

Another procedure you might read about is the resection of Hunner's ulcers in the bladder. Though I was doing 20–25 cystoscopy procedures per week, I only saw Hunner's ulcer a few times per year. When I resected the ulcers, half of the patients were markedly better and half saw little improvement. Despite many years of diligent study, I could not predict who would benefit and who would be made worse by surgery. In my later years, I used surgery when nothing else worked. I am aware that my recommendations may be contrary to current best practices recommendation. This book is about my personal experience and is by no means the final word on anything.

The most respected IC expert in the world, at one point in his career, strongly suggested potassium sensitivity testing in his textbooks on the topic. The test involves putting potassium chloride in the bladder via a catheter. The inventor thought it diagnosed IC. I thought it showed the bladder was sensitive, which we already knew.

Despite the test being our number one diagnostic tool, I stopped doing it in the early 1990's. After I observed women cry and scream in pain after the test, I decided it served no purpose. It never changed the treatments I offered and I viewed it as useless torture. My opinion was in the minority, but if a test did not change what I had to offer the patient, I didn't do it, particularly if it was painful.

PRESCRIPTION DRUG TREATMENTS FOR FREQUENCY, URGENCY, AND PELVIC PAIN SYNDROMES:

- Phenazopyridine (Pyridium, AZO) helps bladder pain, but is not meant to be taken every day for long periods. Most of my patients had already tried the drug before they saw me.
- Methenamine containing drugs (Uribel, Cystex, Urimax, Urogesic, and Urex) contain a mild antibacterial, antispasmodic, and topical analgesic.
- Elavil (generic amitriptyline hydrochloride) worked great for my patients. I first saw it used for phantom limb pain after leg amputation when I was a surgery resident at the VA hospital in Biloxi. The drug works on the chemicals noradrenaline and serotonin to lower the pain stimulus to the brain. It has many potential side effects and must be administered under the care of a doctor who knows your entire medical history. If used in low doses in the right patient, it can be quite helpful. Be aware that it takes up to six weeks to take full effect, and makes some patients sleepy. By the time that the patient gets good pain relief, the somnolence side effect usually has abated. I used Elavil in low doses (10-25 mg. at night).
- Elmiron-pentosane polysulfate (100 mg. every eight hours on an empty stomach) is to my knowledge the only FDA approved drug for bladder pain, at the time of this writing. It is thought to rebuild the bladder lining. The process is microscopic so I don't know if it does this or not. To me,

it seems to decrease inflammation. It must be taken on a strict schedule and on an empty stomach to be effective. In my practice, the drug helped less than 50% of my patients.

- Intravesical therapy involves placing drugs directly into the bladder via a catheter through the urethra. The theoretical advantage is that high levels of medication are delivered into the affected area with fewer systemic side effects. I had much success with the RESCUE cocktail (lidocaine, sodium bicarbonate, heparin, gentamicin), but your specialist will follow the latest research and possibly suggest a different instillation.

- Hydroxyzine hydrochloride (Atarax or Vistaril). Patients took a small dose of 10-25 mg. at night.

- Compounded drugs: As the costs of medical care escalated, I sought ways to decrease patient costs, including teaching selected patients to perform their own intravesical therapy at home. Compounding pharmacies prepared the ingredients as needed. The patients learned to catheterize themselves and instill the agents in their bladder at home after we'd observed success in the office.

- Compounded valium vaginal/rectal suppositories in patients with a spastic pelvic floor or in people who temporarily were worsened by intense pelvic floor manipulation (trigger point release). After their PT appointment, they'd go home and put the suppository in their vagina or rectum and take a 20-minute warm bath. The most effective suppository was B&O (belladonna alkaloid-opium) 30–60 mg. compound. Urologists have used this product to stop bladder spasms post-operatively for decades. It works beautifully but the cost became prohibitive in the outpatient setting. Even though it is a narcotic, I never witnessed addiction or abuse issues with the suppository.

- **Avoid oral narcotic pain medications!** Narcotics are excellent in controlling acute pain after surgery but are not designed for chronic pain management except in terminally ill patients. My experience has been that narcotics, when taken chronically, seem to upregulate the pain receptors until eventually the patient cannot take enough narcotic to dampen their pain. If you need narcotic pain medicine, I strongly suggest you go to a pain clinic run by pain management specialists. The reputable clinics do not advertise on billboards and are not in strip malls with many out of state license plates in the parking lot. Your urologist, gynecologist, or general practitioner should not give you repetitive narcotics prescriptions unless you are on hospice care and expected to die. They should, however, know a reputable pain management clinic in your area.

NEUROMODULATION

Neuromodulation involves alteration of nerve activity using an electrical stimulus. It can be done either peripherally with percutaneous tibial nerve stimulation (PTNS) or centrally with sacral nerve stimulation.

In PTNS an acupuncture-type needle is placed above the ankle and the area is stimulated every week for six to 12 weeks in the doctor's office. An exciting new technology based on peripheral stimulation is mentioned later (eCoin).

Central or sacral stimulation is an outpatient procedure done through a small incision in the upper buttocks to directly stimulate the nerves to the pelvis. The technologies work best in patients with frequency, urgency, or urge incontinence as their primary complaint. In my experience, the types of neuromodulation used in urology were ineffective for pain management alone. However, they were still helpful because if the patient did not have to get up every 30 minutes at night to empty their bladder, they slept much better and the sleep helped them to cope with the pain. Even though the technology is in widespread use and I used neuromodulation for over twenty-five years, we don't know precisely how it works for the bladder. What we know is that it *changes the nerve impulses.*

To further muddy the waters, my observations over the years were: If you had trouble emptying your bladder, neuromodulation helped. If you couldn't hold your bladder, neuromodulation helped. If you had constipation, neuromodulation helped. If you had fecal incontinence or urinary incontinence, neuromodulation helped. If you had diarrhea, neuromodulation helped.

My patients kept detailed diaries about their symptoms and I was always shocked that 25% seemed to get no benefit from neuromodulation, no matter their symptoms and 75% improved no matter their symptoms. From what I know of science and biology, this makes little sense. But, these are my findings from my long clinical experience. I also found very few side effects with these treatments. Neuromodulation was remarkably safe. More about this topic is included in the chapter on incontinence.

OTHER EFFECTIVE PROCEDURES:
- Pudendal nerve blocks benefited some patients. Pudendal neuralgia occurs in patients who sit or ride bicycles for prolonged periods. If you have pelvic pain and cycle, stop cycling for a few months to see if it helps. If you sit most of the day, get a standing desk and a gel seat. The pudendal nerve comes from the sacral area, runs through the pelvic

floor, and ends in the genitalia. It controls many functions and I was unwilling to block a nerve that controlled innervation to the clitoris and penis. Some patients received pudendal blocks from other doctors and had amazing results, but some patients' pain did not improve. If you choose this route, know that the doctor's experience is important. An interventional radiologist may be the best doctor for this procedure in some areas of the country.

- Botox to the perineal muscles improves patients who were recalcitrant to PT and helped with frequency, urgency, and urge incontinence. In the past ten years, Botox has been injected nearly everywhere. When it first came to market, I read *botulinum toxin* and thought injecting it anywhere was a bad idea. I was wrong. It took seven years for me to get on the bandwagon. When I saw it was in widespread use with very minimal side effects, I was astounded. I started using it in the bladder around 1998, doing the procedure in the office. It helped many of my patients, and the only side effects I ever experienced were the occasional patient with urinary retention (it worked too well) and bleeding from the injection sites. Botox wore off in most patients after six to twelve months and needed yearly injections.

- Psychiatric care was the most necessary treatment that I could rarely convince a patient to try. There is still stigma around psychiatry, but for chronic pelvic pain, psychiatric care is imperative. The psychiatrist is the expert in the latest medications that help with the poor sleep, anxiety, depression, fear, and trauma that are part and parcel of this chronic disease. The medications are complex and affect many systems in the body. Like any chronic illness, pelvic pain causes stress at home, at work, and in the individual, which means stress management is crucial. Can you imagine what it's like to be twenty-five years old, be unable to stay out of the bathroom at work, and unable to have sexual activity with your partner? I'd almost never suggest psychiatric care during the first visit because the patient would never come back. Once the patient trusted me, knew I had their best interest at heart, and had tried a few ineffective treatments, they might become willing to consider psychiatric care. Cognitive behavioral therapy greatly helped my patients who committed to it. However, most of my pelvic pain patients would agree to have ten laparoscopies before they would see a psychiatrist. If I could have changed anything surrounding the care of pelvic pain patients, it would have been to find a way to convince them to go to a mental health professional familiar with chronic pain.

Once a year, I dedicated time to read and reread the world's literature on this topic. When I dove deeply into the scientific articles I was impressed with a few things: 1) The problem went away on its own in many patients. You could not figure out what brought it on or what made it go away. 2) Because it sometimes *cured itself*, it was hard to tell if your treatment made it better or if it simply got better on its own. This conundrum serves to further frustrate the patient and make the evaluation of the scientific studies confusing.

Pelvic pain is unlike many other disease processes. Most of the work with pelvic pain is designed to exclude treatable causes and then to manage the symptoms in the least harmful way. I've always felt that no one treatment works well because we are treating multiple problems. Getting a specific diagnosis is the most important step in increasing the chances of good management. I think pelvic pain patients would be best treated in a multispecialty clinic with gynecology, urology, gastroenterology, physical therapy, psychiatry, psychology, pain management, acupuncture, chiropractic care, and hypnotherapy. I've never found a clinic that included all the traditional and non-traditional healing practices in one location dedicated to pelvic pain.

Please know this chapter is about my clinical experience. The gold standard in science and medicine is the randomized, double-blinded, controlled study done with large numbers of patients over a lengthy period. My clinical experience is only my opinion. Real science is expensive and very time consuming. Nothing I have said can stand up to the rigorous demands of science. Please remember that there were likely patients who decided I was not the right doctor for them and went elsewhere. This fact makes my long-term follow up sketchy. This happens with every clinician and certainly happens more often when the available treatments have only a two-thirds chance of helping. I have no long-term follow-up information on the people who left my practice. So please use my opinions to help educate you and help formulate questions for your specialist who knows you best.

IC101–It's Not Just a Bladder Disease by Jill Osborne and Gaye and Andrew Sandler is a wonderful book packed with information to help patients help themselves. A list of links to further assist you is located on the resources page of my website.

Chapter V
Urinary Tract Infection

"Medicine is a science of uncertainty
and an art of probability."
– SIR WILLIAM OSLER

All day long women ask me, "Why am I getting urinary infections?" I always think, but never say, "I wish I knew." Treating urinary tract infections (UTIs) has given me humility.

One in four women has repetitive UTIs. Every few years I search the world's scientific literature for something novel to help these patients. Every decade I find new information that looks promising.

The perplexing question is *why doesn't every woman get bladder infections?* The designer of the female anatomy placed a high concentration of bacteria in the rectum. Much of our amazing microbiome calls this area home. That same creator placed this bacteria-laden organ adjacent to the vagina. A more perfect culture medium for bacteria and fungus could not exist; the vagina is warm, moist, and cozy. The bugs love it. Adjacent to the vagina is the bladder. And, as if this anatomic configuration was not bad enough, the bladder is sterile in many. Some women have bacteria happily living in their bladders. But, for some of the population, the bladder is a sterile organ.

I'm assuming God has better ideas than me. So I'm certain there is good reason for this set up. I view it as excellent evidence that our creator must be a guy. The male urethral opening is 15 to 20 inches away from the rectal opening. That's a long distance for a bacterium to travel. As a result, male UTI is rare. If we had set out to commit bioterrorism against all of womankind, we could not have chosen a better setup.

Enough of my tongue-in-cheek silliness…

WHY DON'T ALL WOMEN SPEND THEIR LIVES IN A UROLOGY OFFICE?

- By drinking fluids, particularly after sexual activity, the mechanical action of the urine flow might wash some of the bacteria out before they can set up a home in your bladder.
- Regular bowel movements without diarrhea or constipation might keep the amount of bacteria hanging around on your perineum (the skin between the back of the vagina and the rectum) lower. ALWAYS WIPE FROM FRONT TO BACK!
- When we are young, the vagina pH (degree of acidity or alkalinity) is maintained by the hormone estrogen. The relatively acidic pH of youth helps avoid urinary infections.
- Emptying the bladder completely correlates with fewer infections.
- The absence of congenital anomalies (inherited anatomic problems) of the kidneys, ureters, bladder, and urethra predicts fewer infections.

- Local immunity factors in the area of the urethra and bladder neck have impact.

I have my suspicions of other factors that keep women out of the urology office. None of the following ideas are *scientifically proven*. No randomized, double-blinded, placebo-controlled studies (RDBPC) exist that I could find.

The purpose of an RDBPC study is to remove the bias of the people doing the study. Random means nobody involved in the study can pick the patients that are most likely to succeed. All patients meeting the study entry criteria are divided randomly into the study group and the control group. The purpose of the control group is to have a group who receive placebos to make sure folks are not getting better simply due to the placebo effect (which is approximately 30% in most studies). The placebo response is complex. The simplest explanation is that in any drug study, around 30% of patients often report *getting better* even if given no treatment. Double-blinded means that neither the person doing the study nor the patient enrolled in the study knows which group they are in. Neither the doctor or nurse, nor the patient knows who is getting treatment and who is on placebo. RDBPC studies serve to keep everyone "honest," but are very expensive to conduct.

To illustrate the importance of this type of RDBPC study, I'll discuss a study I participated in to determine if one overactive bladder drug worked better than another. The study took place at multiple facilities all over the country. We noticed when we compiled the data that at one site, patients were experiencing greater symptom improvement than at all the other facilities. When we drilled down into the details, we found that facility had a particularly lovely and kind nurse collecting the data. Universally, the patients wanted to please the nice nurse and not disappoint her.

When recording their voiding diaries, the patients reported doing slightly better than they were actually doing. The nurse was also inadvertently teaching the patients how to do a bladder drill that helped them. We had to exclude that site from the final data.

This is a simple example of bias. It is human nature that patients want a treatment to work and doctors want their pet project to be helpful to their patients. Science involves taking out as much bias as possible. This example demonstrates that with even the most rigorous application of scientific method, bias can still occur.

What follows is my **opinion** about what contributes to chronic urinary infections and what helps prevent them. My opinion is biased by my experience.

- STRESS, whether perceived as good or bad, gets us out of our routine and causes the body to secrete cortisol. Our immune system defenses are dampened and we become more vulnerable to all types of infections. Often I'd interview patients who had gone on their dream vacation or gotten married or graduated from graduate school or gotten their dream job and also got a urinary infection. My days were full of anxious women worried that their vacations would be ruined by another bladder infection. Stress management is a part of preventing urinary infections.

- Diet could contribute. Brightly colored fruits and vegetables and quality proteins are the building blocks for our immune system. If most of us ate according to the DASH diet (Dietary Approaches to Stop Hypertension), our immune systems might work better. When young women go to college, their diet is no longer the good food served by mom but is often pizza and beer, and they visit me more frequently. Increased sexual activity in these women may be part of the equation, but not always. A high-sugar diet, even without diabetes, correlates with increased incidence of UTI.

- Fluid intake may contribute. Just as there is an appropriate amount to eat for your size body, there is an appropriate amount to drink. Most people who consume more than 1.5–2 liters of fluid per day are hydrated. In our current culture, however, people are being taught to drown themselves. I see five-foot tall women drinking two gallons of water per 24 hours because their trainer told them to. The urinary tract is lined by smooth muscle, has the characteristic of peristalsis (moving boluses of fluid along by squeezing), and can't function as efficiently when it receives too much fluid in too short a time. The kidneys, ureters, and bladder, become dilated and cannot empty effectively. Poor emptying is a risk factor for UTI.

WHAT DO I RECOMMEND?

- If you have fever, chills, blood in your urine that you can see with the naked eye, uncontrolled diabetes, confusion, or flu-like symptoms, go to your doctor or urgent care clinic or the emergency room posthaste.
- If your only symptoms are urgency, frequency, or burning with urination, consider drinking a large glass of water and taking one over the counter phenazopyridine pill and one extra-strength acetaminophen (as long as you are not allergic and have no contraindications to these medications). If your symptoms do not improve in 12 to 24 hours, see your doctor for a urine culture.
- If you are a female and have more than three urinary tract infections in one year, you should consider seeing a urologist.

- If you are a male and have any urinary infection, you should see a urologist. Urinary infections in men are rare and suggest an underlying problem.
- After you have been evaluated by urology to be certain you have no anatomic problem, begin a prevention program and ask to be started on a self-start regimen. This program is discussed in detail later in this chapter.

PREVENTION:
- Drink on average 50–60 ounces of fluid per 24 hours. Avoid any beverage with sugar. Your urine should be pale yellow if you are properly hydrated; unless you are taking vitamins or supplements that can color your urine. You may need more or less fluid depending on your height and your physical activity level.
- If you experience diarrhea, constipation, or fecal incontinence, your gastroenterologist (GI) or primary care doctor can assist. For simple constipation in someone who has had a normal colonoscopy, I suggest polyethylene glycol, 17 grams in 10 oz. of warm water an hour before bedtime. If your stools become too loose, use it every other night or every third night.
- Everyone should know that the chronic use of antibiotics is not healthy. Probiotics can help combat some of the problems with antibiotics. If your gastroenterologist has no suggested program for you, I suggest VSL-3 packets, Visbiome, or Culturelle every 12 hours when you are NOT on antibiotics. I've tried many products over the years and these have proven most effective at preventing bladder infections. Many of my patients have enjoyed normal bowel movements for the first time in years when

they start taking probiotics. Occasionally the probiotic causes excess flatulence, bloating, or diarrhea. If you are in that small group, try using the probiotic every third day. Always follow the advice of your gastroenterologist over anything I suggest.

- Consider taking a quality cranberry supplement every night if you have the occasional UTI or every 12 hours if your infections are recurrent.

- In my experience, the less expensive cranberry supplements are not standardized well enough to be consistent. Many of the cranberry products with the biggest sales budget do **not** contain much or any of the active ingredients that help prevent urinary infections. The supplement industry does not ensure that you get, in all products, what is needed to prevent UTIs. A good quality cranberry supplement cost approximately $1.25 per day in 2022. Buyers beware of the inexpensive cranberry products! You may be getting a deal on something that will not work. The products I recommend are Ellura, Theracran, and Utiva. They contain proanthocyanidins (PACs) that interfere with the bacteria's ability to stick to your bladder wall by exhibiting antiadhesion activity (AAA). There is discussion in the basic science literature about whether pure cranberry juice-derived products or juice plus pomace (seeds, skins, stems of the cranberry) is the best. On my website are a few links if you want to delve further into this matter. Here, I chose to recommend the products that I'd found to be most helpful clinically. I find 36 mg. of PACs in a cranberry supplement taken after dinner, or every 12 hours, to be most effective in decreasing the number of urinary infections per year that occur in an otherwise normal female. The supplements do **not** treat bladder infections. I suggest their use as prevention only. As with all supplements and vitamins, make sure your primary care physician knows you are taking the drugs and approves.

WHY WOULD A CRANBERRY SUPPLEMENT DECREASE BLADDER INFECTIONS?

The proanthocyanidins in cranberries inhibit E. coli from sticking to the bladder wall (decreased bacterial adherence). Since the '80s, patients have told me anecdotal stories of crushing fresh organic cranberries, drinking voluminous amounts of cranberry juice, and taking every type of cranberry supplement. The results were unimpressive in most patients. But occasionally, someone would tell a story lending credence to the idea that cranberry use as prophylaxis against bladder infection might work.

The proper dose of proanthocyanidins was not known. Studies have since shown that 36 mg. of type A PACs every 12 hours does decrease UTIs. However, most cranberry supplements do not contain a standard dose of PACs in each pill. This lack of standardization has led many to believe cranberries don't work. With daily use of a good quality product, my patients' incidence of recurrent UTI with E coli has gone down at least 50%.

Pure cranberry juice (27% cranberry) with no added sugar is effective when ½ cup is ingested every 12 hours. The problem with the juice is weight gain. Over the course of a year, the average woman might gain 10–13 pounds drinking one cup of cranberry juice per day. If you want to decrease your daily calories to accommodate the extra ones from the juice, and you like the taste of cranberry, it will work for you. In 2022, pure cranberry juice sold for around $5 for 32 oz. This put the cost at approximately $1.25 per day, which is consistent with the cost of a good cranberry supplement. I don't fully understand why the pills seemed to work better than the juice in my patient population. Perhaps the patients weren't diligent in drinking the juice. But to me, the calories alone are a good enough reason to go with the pills.

I spent an entire week reading the latest literature on the use of cranberry for UTI prevention. Quite frankly, it gave me a headache. The cranberry supplement industry in the United States is a $90 million per year industry. When considering all cranberry products, the $300 million mark is easily reached. Needless to say, the producers have lobbyists and researchers, and lots of companies are seeking market share. If you want to get a headache too, read the studies I've placed on my website regarding the research. I have not been able to find any head-to-head study involving the supplements that I used for years in my practice. Each has its own marketing points. For the consumer, I'd suggest being sure the supplement has at least 36 PACs per pill. You do not want to purchase an inexpensive pill that does not contain what it should. The marketing on these products is scary.

Cranberry does not treat UTIs, but rather is one way to help prevent them. Prevention is of utmost importance as more and more resistant bacteria develop and we reduce antibiotic use to prevent deaths from resistant bacterial UTI.

When considering options for using cranberry for UTI prevention, make sure you are aware that diabetics, patients on blood thinners, and kidney stone formers need special consideration in their choices. Some products are approved in these special circumstances and some are not. The research is ongoing. Use caution when making your choice.

If you are diligent with my prior suggestions and continue to have more than two infections per year, I suggest you be fully evaluated.

WHAT DOES *FULLY EVALUATED* MEAN TO A UROLOGIST?

- Thorough physical examination of your urethra, vagina, rectum, and if male, your penis
- Office urinalysis
- Possibly catheterized specimen directly from the bladder with post-void residual measurement
- Culture and sensitivity test
- Possible vaginal culture
- Renal ultrasound
- Bladder ultrasound
- Kidney, ureter, and bladder X-ray (KUB) to look for kidney stones
- Possible CAT scan
- Blood work to evaluate renal function
- Possible cystoscopy
- Possible infectious disease doctor consult
- Possible gynecology consult

The bacteria causing a UTI may originate in the kidneys, even though most bacteria come from the rectum. The doctor will begin your evaluation by reviewing all prior cultures to study the type of bacteria in your urine and decide what testing would be most informative. We might start with renal and bladder ultrasounds to look for kidney stones or congenital anomalies causing poor drainage of the urinary tract, and to be certain your bladder empties after voiding.

Kidney stones may be asymptomatic. I have seen patients whose stones filled most of the inside of a kidney yet reported no symptoms. The pain most people associate with kidney stones occurs when a small stone passes down the ureter and becomes lodged. If you have a history of kidney stones, your doctor may order a KUB. This is a low radiation, inexpensive study able to demonstrate calcified kidney and bladder stones.

If you have a significant amount of blood in your urine, have fever or flu-like symptoms, a CAT scan is the most informative radiology test.

I suggest a urine culture when the office urinalysis is abnormal. The culture shows the type of bacteria (E. coli, Klebsiella, Staph., Strep., Pseudomonas, and Proteus) and the sensitivity informs us of the antibiotic most likely to kill it. Commonly used antibiotics are sulfa, nitrofurantoin, penicillin, aminoglycocides, and quinolones. Culture and sensitivity take several days to obtain but is the only way to know precisely what bacterium is present and which antibiotic is most effective.

When your primary care doctor explains that your office urinalysis *appears infected,* they mean that the chemical analysis and microscopic examination of your urine are consistent with UTI. White blood cells, bacteria, and blood suggest you might have a bladder infection. But, until your culture and sensitivity test is completed, days later, your doctor cannot be certain.

In female patients, it is frequently difficult to distinguish between vaginal and bladder infections. Vaginal infections can cause bladder symptoms and bladder infections can cause vaginal symptoms. If the patient has vaginal discharge, it is evaluated also. If we get repeated contamination from vaginal bacteria in our cultures, a tiny catheter is placed through the urethra into the bladder to obtain a more accurate culture.

Blood work is important to determine kidney function. The dose, duration of use, and type of antibiotic are influenced by kidney function.

Cystoscopy is infrequently used in diagnosing the source of UTI. It is helpful if the patient has blood in the urine or is a male with an enlarged prostate. In this procedure, a small flexible scope is passed through the urethra into the bladder. Cystoscopy can be done in the office with local anesthesia or under sedation in an outpatient setting. Bladder stones, bladder diverticula (pouches off the bladder wall), and bladder cancers are easily eliminated as causes of blood in the urine with cystoscopy.

Consultation with an infectious disease doctor is necessary when the patient is growing bacteria that can't be killed by oral antibiotics. In this scenario, intravenous antibiotics are ordered. Patients with multiple drug allergies may be required to see infectious disease doctors to find drugs compatible with their allergy profile. Infectious disease doctors are specialized internal medicine doctors, not surgeons like urologists, and are very helpful when managing sick patients with multiple medical problems in the hospital setting.

Consultation with gynecology is useful when the bacteria grown in culture are typical vaginal pathogens. Urinary and vaginal infections are seen by urology and gynecology alike.

What happens when the patient has had a full urologic evaluation, everything is normal, and the infections persist? Now we're getting to the art of medicine. Traditional medicine suggests the female patient comes to the doctor's office every time she has symptoms of a UTI, gets a catheterized urine culture, and the doctor treats the infection with culture specific antibiotics.

In real life, this does not work! If we always followed this care plan, busy women would be breaking into pharmacies like the storming of the Bastille trying to get antibiotics. Can you imagine a businesswoman traveling internationally with a UTI? She's miserable on a long flight, she finally lands, searches for a doctor in a foreign country, they send a urine culture, she waits for antibiotics, and tries to give her presentation while running to the bathroom every fifteen minutes to urinate blood.

We have overused antibiotics in America. We have caused superbugs with our overuse. But, what else could we do?

If you are drinking appropriate amounts of fluid, taking Ellura, Theracran or Utiva every night, using an excellent probiotic, managing stress, getting adequate sleep, and eating a good diet, you are going to decrease urinary infections by 30% to 70%.

IF YOU ARE FOLLOWING THIS PROTOCOL, HAVE BEEN EVALUATED BY UROLOGY, AND STILL HAVE UTIS, CONSIDER TRYING:

- Topical vaginal estrogen (peri and post-menopausal female)
- Hiprex (methenamine hippurate): One gram per 12 hours
- Vitamin C: 500 mg every 12 hours
- D-mannose: One gram every 12 hours
- If it ever becomes available in the United States, the vaccine for UTI prevention
- Self-start, short term, antibiotic therapy
- Pyridium, acetaminophen, ibuprofen
- Vaginal suppositories of Lactobacilli
- Losing weight if your BMI is over 30
- Avoiding spermicide jelly for birth control
- Other herbal products

To my knowledge, no large RDBCS have been done on these agents. How *might* they work?

Topical vaginal estrogen in the post-menopausal female has been studied in the laboratory and the rat model, and it increases the production of natural antimicrobial substances in the bladder. The tissues also became stronger as topical estrogen seemed to help close the gaps between the cells lining the bladder. This action made it harder for the bacteria to penetrate deeper layers of tissue. Topical estrogen also decreases the shedding of vaginal cells and lessens atrophy.

Topical vaginal estrogen makes the vagina more acidic like it is in younger women. It increases levels of lactobacillus, which is normal flora for the vagina, and correlates with a decrease in pathogenic bacteria.

Estrogen pills, patches, and injections in post-menopausal women may contribute to increased risk for breast cancer and cardiac disease, according to some authors. My reading of the medical literature has not led me to that conclusion. Personally, I think the case for the dangers might be overstated. However, it is clear that the topical forms of estrogen in cream, gel, estrogen rings, and vaginal suppositories, when used in small doses in the vagina, do not appear to have the same risk as the systemic forms of estrogen.

After receiving the approval of my gynecology colleagues, I have used topical vaginal estrogen two to three times per week on thousands of patients and gotten great results. This alone decreased the incidence of bladder infections by half in the post-menopausal female. The main barriers to this treatment in my patients have been fear of hormone use, the cost of care, and *forgetting to use it since use is not every day.*

My thoughts about topical vaginal estrogen and its risks are: How *healthy* are the antibiotics when taken four to 10 times per year? What are those antibiotics doing to your microbiome? Given that your body's cells may be half bacterial; do we really want to murder bacteria in our microbiome that likely function to help us? We know the bacteria that normally live on your body help your body in many ways. How toxic will intravenous antibiotics be when the UTI bacteria are resistant to oral antibiotics and you must take intravenous ones?

I suggest post-menopausal women with recurrent UTI consider topical estrogen unless your gynecologist, oncologist, or hematologist disagrees.

Some of my gynecology colleagues have been doing procedures in their offices to *rejuvenate the vagina*. I have no experience with these procedures and do not know if they help urinary infections or not. The procedures seem to have in common the use of heat energy (laser) to cause tissue to regrow. Many of my patients reported improvement with painful intercourse, vaginal dryness, urinary incontinence, and frequency. If you choose to investigate this technology, be sure you go to a gynecologist who has performed many of these procedures. Any new procedure requires a learning curve and you want an experienced doctor. I could not find a well-done study showing the effects of these procedures in preventing urinary infections. Work in this area is ongoing.

Hiprex or methenamine hippurate is a urinary anti-infective oral medicine. It is an antibiotic but is too weak to use for active infections. It stops the growth of bacteria in urine and can be used as a prevention agent against some but not all bacteria. When the urine is acidic, the drug turns into formaldehyde in the urine and kills bacteria; otherwise it does not work well. Taking vitamin C or decreasing foods that alkalinize your urine can increase effectiveness.

I use methenamine hippurate as a third line of prevention because the side effect profile is high. Many of my patients experienced nausea, abdominal cramping, and diarrhea, and some experienced increased burning with urination while on the drug. Do not take it if you have liver or kidney compromise or are breast feeding, as it does pass into breast milk.

Serious allergic reactions to the medication have never occurred in my practice but have been reported in the medical literature. Since more resistant bacteria are showing up in urine cultures than ever before, I used methenamine more often in the last five years in an attempt to be a good steward of antibiotic use.

Vitamin C has long been thought to help decrease bladder infections by acidifying the urine and making the bladder a hostile environment to some bacteria. Of the two well-done clinical trials I was able to locate, Vitamin C in high doses of 500 mg every six hours did **not** prevent UTI. At these doses, vitamin C is excreted as oxalate, which is one half of the common kidney stone known as calcium oxalate. In one study, taking vitamin C doubled the risk for kidney stone formation in patients who were known stone formers.

My clinical experience suggests the following guidelines for vitamin C use: Use 500 mg of vitamin C every twelve hours to help acidify the urine and increase the effectiveness of methenamine use. Vitamin C alone did little for my patients and was a bladder irritant in many. I suggest that calcium oxalate kidney stone formers avoid high doses of Vitamin C.

D-Mannose has been shown in animal studies to decrease the ability of some bacteria to stick to the bladder lining. In humans, one study using two grams of D-mannose per day for six months showed a 40% decrease in urinary infections during the study period. I have not had those kinds of results. Half my patients report no improvement with D-Mannose and half report a 20% decrease in infections over a year. I made no attempt to control the dose or the quality of the D-Mannose product. I have not seen any ill effects from D-Mannose. One study indicated the D-Mannose attaches to only one type of pili (bacteria "legs" that they use to attach to the bladder) while cranberry PACs attach to several. If you are going to try one pill, use the cranberry first. If you have failed all else, D-Mannose might be worth a try.

VACCINES ARE THE HOLY GRAIL!

Many efforts have been made to develop a dependable vaccine against recurrent urinary infections. I mention a few products, currently NOT available to the general public, to give hope to the person suffering with recurrent UTI. Fear not: lots of smart people are seeking answers in multiple venues.

- EXPEC4V, a vaccine against E. coli, has shown some promise but is still in clinical trials. It is not ready for FDA approval for the general population as of early 2022.
- Uro-Vaxom is a daily oral capsule containing 18 E. coli strains of bacteria. This product is in clinical trials in Germany.
- Urovac is a vaginal suppository containing 10 types of bacteria known to infect the bladder. It has shown some promise in UTI prophylaxis. There are several types of vaginal suppositories being studied around the world. To my knowledge, none are widely available yet.

I mention these currently unavailable treatments to suggest you watch the news for novel ones. Most doctors realize the bacteria are smarter than us and are ahead of the game due to our antibiotic overuse.

SELF-START THERAPY

My patient population is busy. They don't have time to run to the doctor every time they get a UTI! Since 1992, I have been giving patients who are fully utilizing all preventive measures, who are intelligent and in touch with their bodies, three-day or single-day antibiotics to use from one to three times per year if they are not able to come in for a urine culture. Patient satisfaction with this mode of therapy has been very high. I have always worried about causing resistant bacteria, but that does not seem to have happened with most patients on the protocol. After many years of my using common sense to solve a very common problem, the science has caught up.

The Infectious Diseases Society of America and the European Society for Microbiology and Infectious Diseases now suggest:

- Nitrofurantoin monohydrate 100 mg every 12 hours for three days
- Trimethoprim/sulfamethoxazole one double strength every 12 hours for three days
- Fosfomycin trometamol: three grams as one dose
- Pivmecillinam: 400 mg every 12 hours for three days

If the patient cannot take any of these drugs, a fluoroquinolone or beta-lactam drug can be used but are not as desirable.

I was very relieved when the science began to support common sense. In the early 90's, I was worried about getting burned at the stake for witchcraft. But I knew my patients with recurrent UTI would pull me off the pyre.

TREATMENT OF ACUTE SYMPTOMS OF BLADDER INFECTION WITHOUT ANTIBIOTICS:

Over-the-counter (OTC) phenazopyridine and non-steroidal anti-inflammatory drugs (NSAID) or acetaminophen have been used with success.

Several excellent studies have shown symptom relief in 50% of patients with use of OTC phenazopyridine. Seventy percent of patients have symptom relief requiring no further antibiotics with use of NSAIDs (ibuprofen). Neither drug kills bacteria. I don't know how they might work but the studies show they do work. Could they be relieving your symptoms while your body's immune system is killing the bacteria? Could you have inflammation masquerading as an infection? Could you have ingested something that irritates your bladder? Without getting a culture every time, we don't know. But, if you have no allergies to these products, they are certainly worth a try. I suggest taking one dose of phenazopyridine with one dose of ibuprofen or extra strength acetaminophen. If symptoms significantly improve, you may avoid antibiotic use. As always, be sure your doctor knows your plan and checks that there are no drug interactions or other side effects.

VAGINAL SUPPOSITORY WITH LACTOBACILLI

Exactly how and why intravaginal lactobacilli might prevent recurrent urinary infection is unknown to me. They might interfere with adherence and colonization of the vagina by urinary pathogens. Some well-done studies show conflicting results with some showing decreased UTIs and some not. I have not embraced this mode of therapy. I have found intravaginal estrogen to be so effective that I have not sought to use another agent. Additionally, my patients will only put so many tablets in their vaginas before they revolt. If you have a strong contraindication to topical vaginal estrogen, these suppositories might be worth a try. Studies are ongoing and the future holds promise.

WEIGHT LOSS

This is such a touchy subject with patients that I frequently "chicken out" and don't discuss it. I've found that everyone who is overweight knows they need to lose weight. However, the scientific literature shows women with BMI or body mass index over

30 have a much greater incidence of urinary infection. To get an idea of your BMI, visit the Centers for Disease Control website or use an online BMI calculator. Or if you are a science geek like me, divide your weight in kilograms by your height in meters squared. My BMI is 26. I'm not in the obese group but am in the *overweight* group. I recommend you consider getting to your normal weight as part of a program to reduce urinary infections.

OTHER HERBAL PRODUCTS

Women with recurrent urinary infections are frequently desperate. Their lives are interrupted and inconvenienced. When I open the exam room door and see a person with a huge bag full of supplements, I know I am dealing with desperation. Apple cider vinegar, garlic pills, oregano oil, clove oil, myrrh oil, turmeric, CBD oil, uva ursi leaf, marshmallow root and yarrow blossoms, cramp bark tincture, wild yam tincture, and kava are a few of the many products I've seen used.

I have no knowledge of any of these products being studied scientifically for bladder infections. I cannot comment on what they might or might not do. I suggest you follow the things that have been shown to prevent UTI and save these products for future study. Be aware that no matter how *natural* a product might be, it still is foreign to your body and must be processed by your liver and kidneys the same way a prescription drug is processed.

One thing I know for sure is that when patients appear in the office with bags of supplements, we are not doing a good job with that particular disease process.

A SPECIAL CASE OF UTI: GERIATRIC AND MEMORY-CHALLENGED PATIENTS

I almost left this section out of the book. There is little science in what I'm about to tell you. But a dear friend of mine who is a great doctor called me this morning. She was near tears and begging for advice for her beloved mother, who is in the early stage of dementia. She's still able to live at home with the constant care of adoring relatives, but her memory and ambulation are impaired.

My doctor-friend told a tale of woe that I've heard a thousand times. Her mom became acutely confused, was admitted to the hospital to be checked for a stroke or heart attack and was found to have a urinary infection. The mother, despite the best of medical care, was very sick from the infection and was greatly diminished in her capabilities after the experience.

My friend, her very concerned daughter, said, "I'm realistic. I know Mom is on a downward spiral. But I want to keep her out of the hospital and at home as long as we can. I don't want to put her in a facility until I am forced to because I don't want myself and my family to miss out on any lucid moments she might have left."

What my friend needs is a less than perfect plan for an unmanageable situation. She knows I "think outside the box," and even though she knows hundreds of urologists, she wants my experience and my intuition for her most loved relative. She already knows what the textbooks tell us to do.

Conventional medicine and science, with those randomized, double-blinded, controlled studies that I mentioned earlier, dictate that she take Mom to the hospital when she gets more confused because we don't know for sure what's causing the confusion. They would dictate that her mother gets a catheterized urine culture and that the attending doctor treats her with culture specific antibiotics. We learned earlier that the culture takes two or three days to grow. Her mother would be given a powerful antibiotic until the culture returned in case she has a hard-to-treat, hospital-acquired infection. This life-saving antibiotic will likely give her diarrhea and make the whole scenario worse but it could save her life. Remember that she has dementia and the hospital is the most confusing place in the world for a dementia patient. So, she will come out of the hospital "worse than she was before," but alive.

I commonly listen to loving family members in this scenario. They cannot understand why we can't stop this cycle in which UTI is likely the most common cause of death in the elderly female with dementia. I watched middle-aged women torn between trying to do everything for their parents while trying to do everything for their children, hold down a job, and take care of themselves. These women were desperate, frightened, and devoted daughters and mothers. They needed a short-term and unconventional answer to a no-win problem.

I won't bore you with the thousands of patient encounters that led me to my suggestions. Some of the things I suggest have come into vogue in the thirty years I've used them. Some are still anathema that would make the infectious disease community groan.

If you are the caregiver for an elderly woman with memory issues, here's what can decrease the visits to the ER and decrease the hospitalizations for IV antibiotics. Bear in mind that these steps are not likely to be found in any textbook. Mine is unconventional but practical advice born out of caregiver desperation:

- Unless your relative has a history of low sodium (hyponatremia) make sure they drink six to eight ounces of water every 8 hours and have them void every four or five hours while awake, even if they don't feel the need to go. Getting an elderly person to drink and void sounds simple, but can be a daunting task. They don't want to do either, but these two behavior modifications will keep the system flushed out.

- After their evening meal, give them one Ellura or Theracran or Utiva. If your relative has diabetes, be aware that their blood sugar can be affected by these products. If you check their blood sugar in the morning and it starts to be higher than usual, discuss this therapy with the primary care doctor. Some supplements do not elevate the blood sugar. Seek those products when possible.

- Make sure a doctor has checked their post-void residual. If they cannot empty most of their bladder contents (down to 100 cc), then these suggestions won't work and they'll need a catheter to help.

- Hygiene is very important. Every night, wash the vaginal area, rectum, and perineum with a mild soap like Cetaphil. Do not scrub the area. Avoid traumatizing the tender skin. Mildly wash and pat dry. Use a skin barrier if there is any incontinence. Aquaphor or Desitin works the best to provide a barrier between the skin and the ammonia in the urine.

- Unless contraindicated, apply a tiny amount of estrogen to the area around the urethra, the inside lips of the vagina (labia minora), and the perineum. When used every other night or at least three times per week, the hormone cream will change the pH of the area and allow for more lactobacilli which help keep the pathogens at bay.

- Oral probiotics have also been helpful. I gave Culturelle or VSL-3 every day or every other day. Rare patients get diarrhea on these products, but most experienced normal bowel movements. My beliefs about probiotics have little scientific basis that I can find, as goes UTI prevention.

I think they might help absorption of the vitamins and minerals in food that supports our immune system. I also believe when taken long term, they help support healthy gut bacteria and decrease the counts of pathogens that infect the bladder. Doctors disagree, but I suggest stopping the probiotic while on a course of antibiotics and resume the probiotic immediately after finishing the antibiotic.

- If the infections continue despite doing all of the above, try a daily low-dose antibiotic. If there are no contraindications, macrodantin (50–100 mg), Bactrim SS, or cefdinir in low doses can be used at night. Avoiding all antibiotics is the best choice because bacteria are brilliant. Every time you expose them to an antibiotic, they will do their best to mutate and become stronger and start the cycle of needing stronger and stronger drugs to fight stronger and stronger bacteria until they mutate into something we can't treat and the bacteria WIN.

My next and last suggestion is repugnant to the infection doctors. But it works. If the patient has repetitively shown that their worsening confusion is due to UTI, try giving one dose of a quinolone antibiotic before rushing to the hospital. In my experience, single dose quinolones knocked out many infections and ended the cycle for a period of time. I used Cipro 500 mg.

There are several reasons that this mode of therapy drives the infection doctors batty. The main reason is that taking the antibiotic before the patient gets a culture will usually make their culture useless and the doctor will be treating blindly. I avoided this by having my patients obtain as sterile a urine specimen as possible, putting it in the refrigerator until they could drop it at a lab where I kept a standing order for them to bring in urine cultures. They'd do this just before taking the Cipro.

I never experienced success with store-bought urine dip sticks. Theoretically, they could be of service but my patients could not determine when they had a UTI by using a home dipstick. This could improve in the future, which would be a big cost saver for health care.

Over the years, I developed many loyal and happy patients, caregivers, and family members who used this protocol in their elderly memory challenged people. The fate of the elderly woman with dementia and recurrent UTI is that one day the system will fail and she will succumb. Still, this protocol gave the patient and the family more time, decreased hospitalizations, and saved energy, costs and the misery of hospitalization. It was never a long-term cure, but rather an imperfect management tool in an impossible scenario.

Helpful links regarding cranberry studies are located on the resources page of my website.

Chapter VI

Urinary Incontinence

"Listen to your patient- he is telling you the diagnosis."
– SIR WILLIAM OSLER

My first television interview as a young doctor was a commercial about adult diapers. I stood in the aisle of a grocery store and pointed out that there are more types of adult diapers than children's diapers. In the 1980's adult incontinence was still in the closet and rarely discussed. Very few doctors ever asked their patients about the problem. There was much shame surrounding incontinence of urine and feces. Since then, many new treatments have evolved and most people can be treated.

Incontinence is the loss of voluntary control over urination or defecation. I will focus on urinary incontinence, but touch on fecal incontinence superficially.

Incontinence causes distress to varying degrees in different people. Some patients adapt to diapers and others are miserable about a few drops of urine in their underwear. Urine has a strong ammonia smell and can be hard to disguise. The emotional distress of never knowing when incontinence will occur takes a toll.

Some believe incontinence is an expected part of aging, and that nothing can be done but to wear adult diapers.

As a doctor, I've been impressed with the fact that untreated incontinence leads to a domino effect of declining health and accelerated aging. When people are incontinent, they usually decrease physical activity and social interaction. They avoid their tennis group. They stop going to church. It can make an otherwise healthy person into a homebody. I cannot begin to tell you of the thousands of patients I've treated who know every bathroom within ten miles of their home and won't go anywhere that a convenient and private bathroom isn't readily available.

For the primary care doctor, it's important to realize that the lessened activity makes it more difficult to manage the patient's diabetes, hypertension, osteoarthritis, and depression. By treating incontinence, a seemingly unrelated problem, we can help the patient become willing to follow an exercise program to improve their overall health.

How to get help? Your primary care doctor is the place to start. They take your history, examine you, and check your urine to screen for other problems. Some folks will have mild urge incontinence as the only symptom of a low-colony-count urinary infection. Pelvic organ prolapse and vaginal atrophy can be causes for mild incontinence that are found by the primary care doctor. If your incontinence is persistent, you'll be referred to an incontinence expert. Most often, that person is a urologist, urogynecologist, or physical therapist with expertise in the pelvic floor. No matter whom you see that person will need to make sure you empty your bladder and be diligent about your urinalysis.

Nothing is more important in discerning the cause of incontinence than an accurate voiding diary. Keep it for three to seven days and take it with you to your first visit. Make columns to include everything you drink with how much and what type of fluid, the time your incontinence episodes occur, whether those episodes come with cough or with an urge symptom, and whether each one was a large volume leak or a few drops. The diary is a simple tool that helps direct your care and measures progress. There are many templates available on the internet by searching *VOIDING DIARY TEMPLATE.*

WHAT CAN YOU TRY AT HOME BEFORE EVER GOING TO THE DOCTOR?

- Avoid diuretic foods and beverages (caffeine, alcohol, lemons, celery, garlic, onions, watermelon, cucumbers, and ginger).
- Avoid supplements that cause diuresis (dandelion extract, horsetail, hibiscus, green tea, nigella sativa, and parsley).
- Measure your fluid intake to be sure you aren't drinking too much (45–60 oz. of total fluid intake per 24 hours). Decrease fluids two hours before going out to avoid being in a situation with no bathroom nearby.
- Attempt double voiding (when you have finished voiding, stay on the toilet for a full two minutes and try to go again. Do NOT strain. Relax your pelvic floor, tilt forward, and sometimes more will be released).
- Most books on incontinence recommend doing *Bladder Training* which is holding your urine by contracting your pelvic floor when you get an urge to go. Some people swear by this maneuver, but in my clinical experience, I've found it to be of little assistance. There is no negative if you try it at home where you can easily wash up and change clothes if you have an accident.

- Scheduled voiding is helpful, particularly in the older person. As we age, our bladder loses some of its sensation. If you had a beverage at 8 a.m., you should try to void by 10 a.m. Even if you do not feel an urge, go in the bathroom and wait patiently to try to urinate with NO straining. The idea behind this tool is to void before the bladder has a chance to empty without your permission.
- Pelvic floor exercises are easy to learn. There are many excellent free websites with videos. I particularly like the Mayo Clinic site. My favorite self-teaching tools are listed on my website resources page.
- Do not practice Kegels while voiding! Many reputable sites tell you to do this but in my experience, it can worsen urge incontinence. The muscle you are trying to exercise is the muscle you use to cut off your stream. Repeatedly exercising that muscle while voiding may induce bladder spasms.
- Avoid devices that ask you to place something between your thighs and squeeze. The muscle that goes around your urethra doesn't attach to your inner thigh muscles. I have not found those devices effective. What is helpful is a device that goes into the vagina around which you can practice contraction. You might find these devices listed as *vaginal cones or vaginal weights.* Squeeze the muscles you use to defecate to find the right muscle or ask your doctor on pelvic examination to show you where the muscles are located.

In the mid 90's I collaborated with a great physical therapist to produce a product we called *Kegel-A-Go-Go.* It was her voice giving my instructions with background music that sounded like the theme from *The Pink Panther.* The recording could be used in the car to assist with practicing Kegels during commutes. It never caught on, but the idea that you can Kegel anywhere and at any time is the truth. Keep in mind that the muscle around the urethra is similar to other muscles It takes four to six weeks of daily work to judge improvement.

If you've tried these at-home remedies, and are not where you want to be, it's time to see a specialist. Your primary care doctor will know the best incontinence experts in your area. If not, the local hospital that treats women during pregnancy should have a list of approved ones, and if that doesn't lead you to an incontinence expert, ask a nurse. They know everybody!

WHAT HAPPENS WHEN YOU SEE THE INCONTINENCE EXPERT?

- They will take a detailed history and review your voiding diary.
- You'll have a pelvic examination to rule out other issues.
- They'll do either an ultrasound or a catheterized urine test to determine your emptying ability.
- They will check your urinalysis for blood and infection. If you have blood in your urine, you MUST see urology to have the kidney, ureters, bladder, and urethra evaluated. Gynecologists are not kidney specialists.
- They might suggest urodynamic testing if your history is complex and you have failed several treatments (more details about this test later).

WHAT TYPES OF INCONTINENCE ARE THERE?

- Stress (SUI): I HATE this nomenclature because patients think "life stress" when they hear it. Stress incontinence means stress to your pelvic floor brought on by coughing, sneezing, lifting heavy objects, bouncing, running, or any other quick motion requiring abdominal contraction.

- Urge incontinence (UI) is when the bladder releases urine right after a feeling of needing to go. This is the person who gets a quick message that it's about to happen, but it occurs before they can get to the bathroom. The UI episode may be a few drops or a gush down your leg.
- Overflow incontinence is when the patient cannot empty and the very full bladder overflows and leaks.
- Functional incontinence is usually a mobility issue. The person simply cannot get to the bathroom in time.
- Neurogenic incontinence was one of my specialties. It is caused by spinal cord injury, spina bifida, diabetes, multiple sclerosis, Parkinsonism, brain and cord tumors, trauma, and many other nerve conditions. These conditions require the expertise of a urologist who does this kind of work all the time. It is complex and fascinating and can be life changing for the patient battling a complicated health issue. The bowel and bladder must be treated with a coordinated plan for the patient's best benefit. Advanced level studies and complex surgeries are sometimes needed. The question you'd ask when making an appointment is: Is your urologist trained in neurourology? Usually the neurology medical doctors or neurosurgeons know who does a good job in your community.
- Mixed incontinence is a mixture of stress and urge and sometimes poor emptying. These patients are a challenge to treat and will usually need flouro-urodynamics for proper diagnosis.

Let's assume you've gotten the right diagnosis. What treatment options are available? Let's refer back to our categories of incontinence and discuss treatment for each type even though many patients have more than one. The most complex forms of incontinence are beyond the scope of this book.

STRESS INCONTINENCE

Stress incontinence is involuntary leakage of urine with coughing, sneezing, straining, or lifting. If the suggestions for self-treatment have failed, your specialist may suggest:

- If incontinence is mild and you desire improved continence for short periods like going to the grocery or to church, you might consider taking a small dose of an over-the-counter alpha agonist drug. Pseudoephedrine (Sudafed) at 10-30 mg an hour before leaving home can be effective. It works to tighten the bladder neck. Even though it is an OTC medicine, it can have side effects and drug interactions. Please discuss its use with your primary care doctor prior to trying it.

- Use an intravaginal device or large tampon. I had many patients who did not leak except while playing tennis or other sports. Many used an intravaginal tampon to elevate and compress their bladder neck and improve their continence. Many devices are offered on the internet, but I never found anything that worked better than a large tampon. Some patients suffered from dry vagina and needed to use a small amount of K-Y jelly or other vaginal moistening agent to comfortably place the tampon. Remember to take it out after activity! Leaving anything in your vagina for prolonged periods without cleaning can lead to serious and sometimes life-threatening infections.

- Some used a combination of the pseudoephedrine and tampon when going out.
- A pessary is a device fitted by your gynecologist, physician's assistant, or nurse practitioner to lift the vaginal walls and sometimes the uterus with pelvic organ prolapse. When properly fitted and cared for, these devices can be very helpful with mild incontinence and the symptoms of vaginal prolapse. If you decide to try a pessary, be aware that it can take a few visits to find the right device for you.

After I first finished my fellowship, even though I was a surgeon, I was excited to offer non-surgical options to my patients. I knew even then that surgery should be the last option for incontinence.

I was new at fitting pessaries, self-taught, and quite frankly, not all that skilled. One of my early patients had given birth to seven children and her vagina was capacious. She left the morning clinic with a "doughnut" type pessary in place and seemed quite happy. After I returned from lunch, I saw her name on my afternoon clinic schedule. When I walked into the room, one of her young sons stood up, handed me the pessary, and said, "Mom is not happy with you. She coughed in the elevator and your doughnut shot out and landed on the foot of the man behind her. It was covered in slime and stuck to his shoe." I was mortified and the mother's face was red. I didn't ask why she wasn't wearing undergarments; things were tense enough. I learned to have the patients walk around the office, bounce around, and cough before leaving, and never had that problem again.

If at-home Kegels have failed, try physical therapy. The physical therapist (PT) trained in pelvic floor therapy is the most valuable member of the incontinence team. I wish every pregnant woman went to PT prior to giving birth. Understanding the complex pelvic floor, using it properly, and exercising the muscles correctly could improve urination and defecation and decrease incontinence in all women, and in men after prostate cancer surgery.

Depending on the state in which you live, and your insurance policy, you might need a referral to PT from your gynecologist or urologist. I advised all patients to try PT prior to any surgical intervention. If you follow this advice, expect to have a vaginal examination at the physical therapist. The muscles surrounding the urethra attach under the pubic bone, so an external exam only gives the PT superficial information.

Urethral plugs have not worked out for my patients. Every day someone would ask, "Why can't I just put some type of plug in the tube coming out of the bladder while I exercise?" It sounds like a simple solution and I have participated in a couple of studies to try it. However, the urethra is sensitive, is easily dilated and gets infected easily. Pain, worsening of incontinence by dilation or enlarging of the urethra, and infection are the reasons the "plug the tube" solution has not been widely accepted to date. When I studied this option, most patients were so uncomfortable with the device that they begged me to take it out before they even left the office. I hope a smart engineer can solve this problem in the future.

Urethral bulking agents have evolved over the last 30 years. They are compounds that a surgeon injects around the bladder neck through a cystoscope to build up or partially occlude the area of the urethra closest to the bladder. Different compounds have been in vogue at different times of my career. It is a simple procedure in the hands of someone who does it all the time. If you choose to try this treatment, be sure your surgeon has done many of these procedures because a few tricks that come with experience can improve the success and diminish the complications of urinary retention and worsening incontinence.

POSSIBLE BULKING AGENTS:
- Autologous fat (your own fat)
- Glutaraldehyde cross-linked bovine collagen
- Calcium hydroxylapatite
- Pyrolytic carbon-coated beads
- Polydimethylsiloxane
- Ethylene vinyl alcohol copolymer
- Dextranomer hyaluronic acid
- Polytetrafluoroethylene

When you see a multitude of products used for a surgical procedure, it usually indicates that there is no perfect treatment. If your surgeon is skilled and experienced, you may enjoy a 70% success rate and likely need repeated injections over time. In my experience, the bulking agents' efficacy lasted one to seven years in most patients.

SURGICAL TREATMENT OF SUI

Surgery has greatly advanced since I became a urologist. The use of vaginal mesh has been controversial, but its use for urethral suspension has been very successful, with low morbidity in the hands of surgeons who do the procedures frequently. No surgery has a 100% success rate. If a surgeon tells you they have a 95–100% success rate with anything, don't believe them. No surgeon can control the way your body heals a procedure.

I remember doing the same procedure on six different women on the same day. Four were typical incontinence patients: average weight, near or early into menopause, and active but not truly athletic. One patient was a triathlete with little body fat and very healthy. My last patient was an elderly woman who was a little overweight and had mild hypertension and well-managed diabetes. The night before surgery, I had worried about the older woman with several comorbidities and questioned my decision to perform surgery on her. I thought if anyone might have trouble it would be her.

At the time, we kept everyone overnight after a pelvic procedure. When I made rounds at 6:30 the next morning, the triathlete was miserable with pain. The catheter had given her extreme bladder spasms which we could never completely control until the catheter was removed. The elderly patient was sitting fully dressed on the side of her bed, impatient to be discharged, because she "had to get to doggy day care or they would charge her another day for her poodle."

Five of the six patients had great outcomes; the triathlete's surgery failed. Every patient received the same procedure with the same surgeon. I gave each lady the best operation I could offer. Over the next ten years I came to realize that even though it was totally counterintuitive, very athletic women seemed to fail incontinence surgery more often than others. I could never prove it, but I felt that because of their very strong abdomen, athletes could generate high vector forces out of their vagina. The vagina is basically a hole open to the ground. If I made the sling around their urethra tight enough to combat the high-pressured cough or sneeze, they'd not be able to urinate and would have urinary retention. I came to this conclusion by viewing the flouro-urodynamics studies of my and thousands of other doctors' patients who had failed incontinence surgery.

Over the years, I came to realize that 15% of my carefully chosen patients would fail my best incontinence procedure and I often never knew why. Occasionally, it was because they refused to follow post-operative instructions to limit activity. Mostly, it was a mystery. I could not correlate age or hormone status or weight or comorbidities to predict success. One of my former nurses used to say, "If Dr. Boone can't scare them off with her statistics, then she'll operate on them." I loved doing incontinence surgery but always said a silent prayer when I saw a post-operative patient on my clinic schedule. I loved the 85% who smiled with gratitude and felt my stomach fall an entire floor when I saw that disappointed look.

Don't be afraid of surgery if you need it. You have an excellent chance it will work. But please, try everything else first.

TYPES OF SURGERY FOR SUI:
- Mid-urethral sling is one of the most common procedures worldwide. It involves placing a narrow strap of synthetic material under the urethra, usually through a vaginal incision.
- Traditional sling is when a longer strip of your own tissue called fascia or synthetic material is passed from a small abdominal incision into a small vaginal incision and back up around your urethra to form a hammock to support the urethra tube. It's usually chosen in more severe cases of incontinence or in repeat surgery where prior incontinence procedures failed.
- Colposuspension is less commonly used. It involves making a cut on the lower abdomen and lifting the bladder neck from inside the body. This procedure can be done during laparoscopy or using open surgery techniques.
- An artificial urinary sphincter is rarely needed in women. This is a complex mechanical device that must be implanted by a surgeon familiar with the procedure. An inflatable

circular cuff is placed around the urethra and attached to a small pump in the labia or scrotum which in turn is attached to a fluid-filled reservoir placed in the lower abdomen. I used these most often in men after radical prostatectomy and in patients with spina bifida or other neurologic disorders. The device works beautifully in the hands of a surgeon who has lots of experience with it.

My practice was based mostly on redoing other surgeons' failures. The first-time surgery is the most likely one to work well. Because of my extra training in reconstruction, I had a five-state referral for the most difficult cases. I was blessed to always work out of world class hospital systems (Tulane Medical Center, University of California-Davis, The Medical College of Georgia, Ochsner Health System, and Northside Hospital-my favorite!) I've always had the great benefit of excellent urodynamic nurses.

Urodiagnostic studies are a group of complex tests and are very operator-dependent. While some doctors do the testing in their offices, I saw more poorly conducted tests from offices than well-done tests. The test involves having small catheters with microchip transducers placed in the bladder and vagina or rectum. The patient is seated on a toilet seat in front of an X-ray table. The bladder is slowly filled with contrast material that is visible under fluoroscopy. The patient is asked to relax (yes, really) as the bladder fills, to cough and strain and attempt to create the conditions under which they leak urine. In the hands of well-trained urodynamic nurses and a doctor who reads the studies well, the test can be a very valuable way to diagnose complex incontinence. Most patients don't need this study prior to treatment. But, if you have mixed incontinence, or have failed surgery or you have neurologic issues, it is extremely helpful. I read five to 15 of these studies every week for 32 years and was a regional expert with referrals from many doctors. It was fascinating to help patients with complex problems and fun to collaborate with smart, motivated nurses.

If you want to read what the doctors read on this subject, The American Urologic Association, The American College of Obstetricians and Gynecologists, American Urogynecology Society and The National Health Service are excellent resources.

Stress incontinence is mostly the purview of the physical therapist and the urologic surgeon or the urogynecologist.

URGE INCONTINENCE (UI)

UI is a strong uncontrollable urge to urinate that one cannot delay, leading to leakage varying from a drop to total emptying of the bladder.

We (urologist, gynecologist, physical therapist, primary care doctor, physician assistant, or nurse practitioner) can best serve our patients with urge incontinence by using a written care pathway for each patient. I was concerned that patients forgot most of what I said and was concerned that many thought if an overactive bladder drug had failed, which most did, that there were no further answers. The written, individualized care pathway aids primary care, the gynecology and urology doctors, but most importantly, our patients. The care pathway would include their current treatment plan, how long it should continue, the interval at which they will be re-evaluated, and the next step if the current plan is not successful.

I think of the plan as a roadmap towards success that the doctor and patient can follow together. The best treatment plan would also include the patient's definition of success. Do they want to *sit through a two-hour movie?* Do they want to *decrease the number of times they void per day to ten?* What are our patients' goals?

CAUSES OF UI:
- Drinking more fluid than your urinary system can handle
- Bladder irritants (alcohol, caffeine, diuretic foods)
- Medications and supplements with diuretic effects
- Chronic constipation
- Aging
- Menopause
- Infection
- Bladder cancer (extremely rare cause)
- Neurological diseases (brain, spinal cord)
- Medical diseases (diabetes, multiple sclerosis, Parkinsonism, stroke)
- Obstruction (prior surgery, urethral strictures, enlarged prostate, severe vaginal prolapse, tumors – again rare)
- Inflammation and scarring
- Bladder stones
- Obesity

HOW MUCH WATER DOES THE BODY NEED?

I practiced the last few years in a very affluent part of metro Atlanta where many of my patients had trainers. It was in vogue for a number of years for the trainers to tell their clients to "drink as much water as you possibly can." Every day I saw women who were five feet tall, weighed 100 pounds, and drank more than a gallon of water per day! I'd perform kidney and bladder ultrasound and find they had given themselves hydroureteronephrosis (dilation of the entire urinary tract) with poor emptying.

Even when I showed them normal studies and compared the normal studies to my patient's studies, they could not accept that their trainer was wrong. When I'd suggest they decrease fluids for two months and do a voiding dairy every week to plot their progress, most would not fully participate. They wanted drugs or surgery for a self-induced problem. I wrote to many *women's* magazines in an attempt to discuss this problem but got NO takers. When the populace wants something to be true, it's hard to buck the belief with facts. The patients brought articles by all kinds of "experts," none of which were urologists and argued the points. Some went elsewhere and never returned. Most returned after trying multiple other drugs and invasive procedures.

To reiterate, at the very most, your body can tolerate your body weight in pounds divided by two as a guideline for the number of ounces to drink in total for 24 hours. Example: 140 pounds / 2 = 70, so at the very most with vigorous exercise and lots of sweating, you can tolerate 70 oz. per 24 hours. Most 140-pound people with a sedentary lifestyle needs approximately 50 oz. per 24 hours. If you have conditions like kidney stones that require you to drink more, then ignore this advice. But, if you are an otherwise normal person and have UI, the first thing to do is make a diary of exactly what and how much you drink per 24 hours. Do this for a week to get the best information for yourself and your doctor.

We discuss getting bladder irritants out of your diet in our chapter on IC. If you are taking a diuretic, do not stop it unless your doctor agrees.

CHRONIC CONSTIPATION

Chronic constipation is a common cause of UI. When the colon is chronically full, it presses on the uterus and bladder. If you have no uterus, the full colon compresses the bladder against the pubic bone and pushes it into the vagina, which can cause bladder spasms. In children and women, improving bowel emptying can cure mild UI. I am not a gastroenterologist so please see your GI about constipation to be certain it's nothing serious.

If your colon has been determined to be normal, you might try the following to improve bowel emptying:

- Exercise
- Increasing fiber (30–40 grams per 24 hours) and monitor water intake to attain approximately 50 oz. of total fluid per 24 hours
- Probiotics (VSL-3, Visbiome, Culturelle)
- Physical therapy (Many women have abnormal voiding and defecation patterns and PT can help.)
- Taking the supplement magnesium citrate at night or every other night. (As with all supplements, be sure your primary care doctor knows and approves.)

If you have tried all of the above and are still having problems emptying your bowel, I suggest:

- Stool softeners (Dulcolax, bisacodyl).
- Osmotic-type laxative (Miralax, polyethylene glycol 3350). I found this product to be the most manageable. I'd have my patients start therapy with half the prescribed dose on the bottle (17 grams of powder dissolved in six oz. of liquid) and do that every third night. Half of 17 grams is approximately half the cap of the bottle. If that didn't work, we'd increase it to ½ dose every other night, then ½ dose every night. If that did not work and the GI doctor was sure the bowel was normal, I'd have my patients move to a full dose every night. I never saw any problems or complications with this plan, even when used long-term.

However, patients who advanced the dose too quickly did experience unmanageable diarrhea. If you need to advance the dose, do it slowly!

- Some patients used glycerin suppositories every morning after a hot beverage to help retrain their bowel.
- Enemas and strong suppositories and oral mineral oil should be last resorts and used with the guidance of your doctor.

OPINION: AMERICAN REASONS FOR BOWEL PROBLEMS

When I've been to international medical meetings and discussed constipation with colleagues, American women seem to have more bowel issues than those in other countries. I believe some of our problem comes from societal norms. Men awaken, drink coffee or tea, and have their morning bowel movement. Women tend to the kids, multitask with home organization, and learn to ignore the "gotta go" message from the lower bowel until it is "convenient" to go. With our very busy lifestyles, the entire day may pass with never a convenient time to have a bowel movement.

I think another issue is that women don't want to stink up a bathroom they share with others. Women don't want to have a bowel movement at work, at their friend's house, or at the club after tennis or yoga. My observations support the idea that women from other countries don't seem to be as self-conscious about natural body odors.

Over the years, our bowel learns we aren't on a regular schedule and dampens down the signal. This is my opinion and is not backed by any scientific study. My opinions are formed from listening to women talk about their bowels for many years.

Many women will improve by simply making a commitment to have a bowel ritual around the same time every day. Watch men…NOTHING gets between them and their time to go! Pick either morning or evening, drink a warm beverage, sit in the bathroom for a few minutes and try to go. Over time, things will usually improve and you might cure two problems with one simple behavior modification.

AGING

In my early years as a urologist, I was taught that the bladder became overactive due to decreasing estrogen with aging. I also was taught that men got UI due to the obstructing and enlarged prostate. When I did voiding diaries on men and women and matched them for age alone, ignoring sex, estrogen status or enlarged prostate, I found that regardless of any other factors men and women had increasing voiding dysfunction due to age. The older they were, the more they suffered. So, the aging bladder is part of the incontinence problem. For a decade I gave the prostate symptom score to women just to see how they scored and amazingly, the women had obstructing prostates too! I say this tongue in cheek because obviously, unless a person has undergone gender reassignment from man to woman, women don't have a prostate. I use this example to further support the idea that UI may be due in part to aging and not necessarily due to a lack of estrogen or an enlarged prostate.

MENOPAUSE

We know that decreasing estrogen levels in the vagina cause changes in the microbiome, which is the normal yeast and bacteria which live in the vagina. These changes lead to increased frequency of UTI and bladder irritability. Some patients only experience UI when they have a UTI.

A decreasing estrogen level leads to the loss of strength in the pelvic muscles and can contribute to UI. It can also lead to thinning of the tissues around the urethra and vagina.

In my practice, I found that applying small amounts of topical estrogen to the vagina every other night greatly decreased the incidence of UTI and UI in post-menopausal women. Please be aware that in most patients, six to eight weeks of diligent use was required before the incidence of UTI decreased and severity of UI improved. Intra-vaginal estrogen use must be maintained to experience continued efficacy. If the patient stopped using it, the problems reoccurred.

When topical estrogen was applied to the vagina for six weeks prior to incontinence surgeries for SUI, the tissues were healthier and the surgery healed better. I believe the estrogen increased blood flow to the tissues.

My favorite estrogen was the Vagifem 10-microgram pellet applied to the vagina every Monday, Wednesday, and Friday night. If this product is cost prohibitive with your drug plan, your gynecologist will know the current best protocol options for you.

CURRENTLY AVAILABLE VAGINAL ESTROGEN PRODUCTS:
- Estrace
- Estring
- Femring
- Ortho dienestrol
- Premarin
- Vagifem
- Compounded vaginal estrogen products
- Generic products

If you read the package insert on estrogen products, you will conclude that your doctor is trying to kill you! But in truth, I never had any problems with any of the products. If the patient had a history of blood clots or breast cancer, I'd always have their doctor approve the use of the product. Most oncology and hematology doctors okayed use of low dose topical vaginal estrogen products. Of course, ALWAYS defer to the judgement of your doctor. These conditions can be serious, and decisions to use or not use estrogen need to be made on an individual basis.

URINARY TRACT INFECTION AND INTERSTITIAL CYSTITIS AS CAUSES OF URGE INCONTINENCE

Inflammation causes irritability, and irritability causes bladder contractions, and bladder contractions cause urge incontinence. I saw many patients who only had UI when they had a UTI or IC flareup. When the IC flare or UTI were properly managed, the incontinence went away. For these patients, I'd make sure they could empty well and then consider using a bladder antispasmodic for a few days for relief. There will be more information about these products in the treatment section of this chapter.

UI was an extremely rare symptom in patients with bladder cancer in my practice. Most patients who proved to have bladder cancer had blood in the urine as their earliest symptom. If you have UI, make sure your doctor checks your urine for blood (hematuria), but don't worry about bladder cancer as your first thought. If the UI persists, you will need to see a urologist and they'll determine if you need to be evaluated for bladder cancer. Remember, most women with UI do NOT have bladder cancer.

NEUROLOGIC DISEASES AND MEDICAL DISEASES

Any condition, disease, or medical problem that affects your nervous system can affect your bladder. The nerves to the bladder begin locally around the bladder, travel through the pelvis into the sacral spinal cord, and travel up to the brain stem and brain. This fascinating highway of complex interactions formed the study of an entire year of my life. Neuro-urology was always my favorite lecture to give to medical students and residents.

The details of the innervation of the urinary tract are beyond the scope of this book. Be aware that knowledge in this field grows every year and our ability to intervene improves. For the purposes of this book, please know that any disease that has the potential to affect the brain, spinal cord, or peripheral nerves can affect your bladder function.

COMMON DISEASES CAUSING UI:
- Diabetes (DM)
- Multiple sclerosis (MS)
- Spinal cord tumor
- Spina bifida
- Spinal cord injury
- Pelvic tumors
- Brain injury and trauma (stroke, closed head injury)
- Parkinson's disease
- Dementia (Alzheimer's)
- Brain tumors
- Pelvic organ prolapse
- Enlarged prostate

If you have any of these problems, please tell your doctor about your incontinence because sometimes by better controlling the underlying disease, the incontinence will improve. For example, I routinely saw patients with diabetes improve their incontinence when their diabetes control was better. One man lost 25 pounds and was able to stop using a diaper. I saw patients with MS and Parkinsonism have their incontinence cured by adjusting their drugs and better managing their primary disease. This list is not inclusive of all diseases that affect the bladder nerves but represents the most common.

URINARY OBSTRUCTION AND BLADDER STONES

The most common causes of outlet obstruction of the bladder:

- In men – urethral stricture or prostate enlargement
- In women – pelvic organ prolapse, scarring from prior surgery, and urethral stricture

Obstruction causes UI by inflaming the bladder. Imagine the bladder fighting to push the urine out past a blockage of some sort. It becomes thickened and irritated. Sometimes if the obstruction is chronic, the patient will have crystals form in the base of the bladder and stones will form on those crystals. Bladder stones usually cause blood in the urine, but occasionally present to the doctor with frequency and urgency. I've taken stones as big as golf balls out of patients who did not know they were in them. The largest stone I ever removed was the size of a baseball, in a man whose prostate was the size of a grapefruit. Large stones are rare findings in modern urology.

In women, I saw on average of once a month someone who had pelvic surgery of some type and a stitch had eroded into the bladder over time. Usually it was from an incontinence procedure, but not always. I had referrals from over three-hundred gynecologists and urologists for their complex incontinence patients. So, bladder stones after surgery are very rare, despite my having seen them often. If you have blood in your urine, you will be sent to urology and suggested for cystoscopy via a small fiber-optic scope, which will detect any bladder stone.

Obesity can cause incontinence. It makes sense that having pounds of internal adipose pressing on the bladder flattens it, making it unable to fill and more irritable. The relationship between obesity and incontinence is complex. I regularly performed flouro-urodynamic testing where we looked at the bladder with X-ray and watched this phenomenon in real time. But there are likely factors we have not discerned, as many obese people have no problem with incontinence. The medical literature lists obesity as a cause of incontinence. Losing weight makes surgery more likely to be successful. I am not certain that losing weight guarantees correction of incontinence.

TREATMENTS FOR UI:
- Kegel exercises
- Physical therapy
- Bladder drill
- Medications
- Neuromodulation
- Onabotulinumtoxina A (Botox) injection

We've covered Kegels, physical therapy, and bladder drill in other sections. There are many drugs that work for this condition. You will recognize some from the advertising. On TV, the drugs have been listed as treating Overactive Bladder (OAB) which is the continuum of frequency, urgency and urge incontinence.

MEDICATIONS FOR TREATING UI:
- Tolteradine (Detrol)
- Oxybutynin (Ditropan)
- Darifenacin (Enablex)
- Fesoterodine (Toviaz)
- Solifenacin (Vesicare)
- Trospium (Sanctura)
- Mirabegron (Myrbetriq)
- Hyoscyamine (Levsin- SL)
- Flavoxate HCL (Urispas)
- Amitriptyline
- Oxytrol patch (transdermal oxybutynin)
- Gelnique topical (oxybutynin gel to apply to the skin)

When you see a long list of drugs treating one condition, it usually indicates: 1) None of the drugs stand out as the best in class. 2) The disease being treated is very common and multiple companies are trying to get market share. 3) The older drugs have too many untoward side effects and each new one has a lower side effect profile and hopefully greater efficacy.

In the spirit of full disclosure, I have given hundreds of talks on incontinence, many supported by industry. By 2000, the pharmaceutical industry was highly regulated in its interactions with physicians, and thus began the era of "direct to patient advertising." In my mind, marketing prescription drugs to patients is not a good idea. Unfortunately, some doctors abused their past relationship with pharmaceutical companies and the government stepped in with what I believe was an even worse solution. We hoped their putting up blockades between the doctors and pharma would decrease drug cost. Unfortunately, the "direct to patient advertising costs" were greater than the "marketing to doctors costs" and prescription drug costs never went down. The cost of prescription drugs is outrageous in our country, but that is a topic for another book.

All of the drugs listed decrease the incidence of pure UI. All of them have side effects. All have drug interactions with other drugs. Each can be safely used in the hands of prescribers who are familiar with this class of drugs and who know all of your medical problems and have a complete list of every medication you take.

In my practice, many patients had unsuccessfully tried tolteradine or trospium or solifenacin before they came to me. Many had not taken the medication long enough. If you choose to take one of the drugs in this list, I suggest you keep a voiding diary, take the drug for an entire month if you have no untoward side effects, and then redo the diary. You and your doctor will get the most information with that plan. If medication has not worked in a month and your voiding diary has not improved, I'd suggest your primary care doctor refer you to an incontinence expert.

Because my patient population was considered complex, my experience was skewed. My favorite OAB medication used to be Ditropan XL. It had a very sophisticated delivery system that decreased side effects and increased efficacy over an 18-hour period. Unfortunately, a competitor had more marketing dollars and my favorite drug went to generic. As a result, the sophisticated delivery system was no longer used and the drug has all the side effects of the parent compound. Dry mouth, dry eyes, constipation, and dry skin are common complaints. Generic drugs can be safe and efficacious but are often NOT biologically the same as the original product due to bioavailability and alterations in the delivery system.

Since my favorite OAB medicine was no longer produced and other drugs had often failed my patient population, I reverted to what I nicknamed *My Best Trick* or Myrbetriq (mirabegron). It was the newest in class, with better efficacy, fewer side effects, and fewer drug interactions. But, it has been expensive on some drug plans. All drugs in this list have to be taken forever to obtain continued efficacy. They do not cure incontinence. They manage it.

I include patch and topical agents that I believe are no longer offered by any pharmaceutical company because they failed to achieve market share. These products can be made by compounding pharmacies if desired.

The idea behind using topical drugs is that by bypassing the digestive tract and liver, the breakdown products that cause some of the untoward side effects are avoided and the first pass effect, where drug concentration is reduced, can be circumvented.

WHAT SHOULD YOU DO?

If you have mild UI, start with the cheapest drug at the lowest dose after your doctor has made sure you empty your bladder well. Try that drug at that dose for a full month before passing judgement.

If you have some improvement and no unacceptable side effects, ask your doctor if you can increase the dose and try the higher dose for one more month. If your symptoms of OAB are still problematic, ask for referral to an incontinence expert. Almost all of these drugs can cause constipation, which will make OAB worse. So, be sure that you are monitoring your bowels and start a bowel program if necessary.

In my long experience with these drugs, less than 50% of people who come to urology can be managed with medicines. Please be aware that the bladder can "downregulate its receptors" so a drug that worked beautifully for years will suddenly no longer work. Your doctor can switch you to another drug with a different mode of action on the bladder for three months and then you can return to the one that worked best. In the general population of the primary care doctor, this class of drugs works to treat UI two-thirds of the time. These drugs are certainly worth trying, but don't be surprised when you need other therapy.

NEUROMODULATION

Neuromodulation is my favorite treatment, besides physical therapy, for UI and OAB (frequency and urgency and urge incontinence). I like it because there are no drug interactions, no allergy to drugs, no constipation issues, no long-term financial expenditure for medication, and it can greatly improve patient symptoms.

What is it? Neuromodulation is the alteration of nerve activity through delivery of a stimulus. In urology, it is the delivery of electrical stimulation to normalize nervous system function. Neuromodulation has been around at least since the 1960s. I saw my first case of sacral neuromodulation for the bladder in 1988. It had been studied for the bladder by several urologists at The University of California, San Francisco around 1982. The technology has progressed greatly over the last forty years. The incisions have gotten smaller, the tests to determine if it might work can be done in the office, and the devices have gotten smaller too. I first used it in 1989 and continued to use sacral neuromodulation routinely with great success.

In the early '60s the cardiac pacemaker came into widespread use. Through innovative biomedical engineering, many lives have been saved. Similar technology was used for the bladder. A small incision is made in the lower back and under fluoroscopic guidance, a tiny electrode is placed near the nerves that innervate the bladder. A small stimulator is placed under the skin and the incision is closed. This is a simple outpatient procedure that is often performed with sedation.

Within a few days, the UI symptoms are improved in 80% of patients. I consider this an extremely good success rate; given that almost all the patients I treated with neuromodulation had failed multiple prior treatments and had worse symptoms. There were very few complications, but infection is always possible with implantation of a foreign body. Again, you want to see a surgeon who does these cases all the time so your operative time is short and they are very familiar with the latest protocols. I always worked with the Medtronic Company and found their continuing education to be helpful even though I had done many implants. Their well-educated and knowledgeable technicians (Interstim therapy consultants) were available to assist me and my patients with any technical matters. I received no financial remuneration from the company for my relationship with them.

Despite seeing amazing results with sacral neuromodulation, it was a hard sell to many patients due to cost and insurance issues. Insurance companies wanted the patients to try many other treatments before they would consider paying for neuromodulation. Also, some patients did not want an implantable device or anesthesia. Unfortunately, the few patients who did experience complications were very vocal on the internet, so others would research the device and scare themselves instead of trusting their doctor. The thousands and thousands of success stories rarely made it to the search engines. Fearmongering has kept many from getting excellent care that could have made their lives so much more enjoyable.

Around 1990, I became very interested in trying to modulate the nerves to the bladder by using the tibial nerve. This involved working with an acupuncturist who was willing to help; with acupuncture alone, we got minor improvements. Later, the technology of percutaneous tibial neuromodulation (PTNM) was developed. In this in-office procedure a tiny needle is placed near the tibial nerve by the ankle. The patient receives 30 minutes of low-level stimulation. My patients needed a total of 12 sessions for full benefit.

During the first year I did it, I did not charge anyone because my experience had not been good with simple acupuncture and I wanted to generate my own data and experience before offering it to my patients. I used the procedure in those who had not improved with conservative treatments and medications and refused sacral neuromodulation. Despite using it in the worse cases, I saw an 80% cure rate in my patients. I never saw any complications other than occasional mild bruising at the needle site. In my experience, if the patient had not seen improvement by the sixth treatment, they did not get it with the last six treatments. But, if they saw improvement by treatment six, and went on to the 12th session, they enjoyed long-term success. I followed the patients for two years after the last treatment. One in 25 patients needed boosters of monthly treatments. I could never determine the characteristics of the patients who needed the booster to continue efficacy.

In Atlanta, coming to the doctor once a week for 12 weeks was a burden to most. Our traffic during work hours (6 a.m.–8 p.m.) is challenging. Many who could have benefitted from this procedure could not participate due to the time involved. This mode of therapy became even more challenging during COVID when office visits were limited.

In 2022, a new and exciting option has come to my attention. The biomedical technology company Valencia Technologies has produced the only FDA-approved implantable tibial neurostimulator that can be placed under local anesthesia in the office. The device is a permanent implant and is suitable for the patient who does not have time for a dozen or more office visits to receive percutaneous tibial neuromodulation or does not want the outpatient surgery for the implantation of the sacral neuromodulator. The eCoin device is implanted via an incision in the lower leg and placed below the skin over the tibial nerve. It is programmed via an external controller.

Comparative studies have not been conducted to determine the relative efficacy and complication rates of different technologies, or which device or procedure works best in which patient. I have been impressed with the success and low complication rate of all the options.

Both sacral and percutaneous tibial neuromodulation were quite popular. The cost of incontinence devices and prescription drugs, as well as the inconvenience of always having to be prepared for a leakage episode, made these treatments cost effective. It is rewarding to help incontinent patients reclaim their lives. The field of neuromodulation is growing and new devices and technologies are being developed. I'm excited about the future in this area!

BLADDER BOTOX (ONABOTULINUMTOXINA A)

I have to admit that I was late to the party in using this form of therapy. One of my most respected colleagues was in on the early studies. I knew her to have great integrity but when she reported results that were too good to be true, I was skeptical. Plus, the idea of using a toxin to treat a disease seemed crazy to me. Bladder Botox had been widely used for seven years before I was willing to try it. I took the *Primum, non nocere* creed to heart: *First, do no harm.*

I'm happy to report that I was dead wrong. Botox has been used by millions upon millions with little trouble. It has been applied to multiple diseases with great clinical benefit to patients.

Once I decided that I had a large patient population for whom all else had failed and would not consent to neuromodulation (my other best trick), I decided to try Botox.

It proved to be an easy in-office procedure with quick results that lasted six to 14 months. It was imperative to be certain the patient did not have a UTI at the time of the procedure and that their blood clotting was normal. It worked so well in my patients that 10% experienced short term urinary retention. It was a miracle drug in spinal cord injury patients who used intermittent catheterization to empty their bladders.

I had the occasional patient who had slight bleeding afterwards. But amazingly, 85-90% were significantly improved or essentially cured until the Botox wore off and it had to be repeated. For reasons I don't understand, Botox seems to be absorbed in other parts of the body at around three months post procedure and needs to be repeated every three to six months. In the bladder, we routinely were able to do the Botox injections every ten to 14 months or approximately once per year in most people. In neurologic patients I used 300 units if they routinely catheterized themselves and in those with no neurological disease I used 100 units to decrease the chances of post-procedure urinary retention.

If you choose this mode of therapy, go to an experienced surgeon. It's a simple procedure, but you want the benefit of an experienced surgeon as excellent technique improves the chances for success.

Nocturia or frequent urination at night is not always a urologic condition. Causes include:

- Drinking too much fluid or diuretic fluids too close to bedtime
- Sleep disorders like sleep apnea
- Poor bladder emptying

- Taking diuretic drugs at bedtime
- Urine infection
- Enlarged prostate
- Poorly controlled diabetes
- Heart disease with leg swelling
- Anxiety
- Overactive bladder
- Neurological diseases

Again, a voiding diary is helpful in discerning the nature of your problem. I'd ask my patients to weigh themselves first thing in the morning and last thing at night and record the numbers. Then I'd have them measure and record everything they drank for each 24-hour period, as well as the time and volume of urination. We provided devices that fit on their toilet to make it easy. (McKesson makes a commode specimen collection device that can be purchased online, if your doctor does not have one.)

If you get up at night to urinate frequently and have any of these symptoms:

- Swollen legs during the day,
- Low urine output during the day,
- High urine output at night after bedtime, or
- Weighing more than two pounds more at night than in the morning, then

See your internal medicine doctor, cardiologist, or nephrologist instead of the urologist. You'll need to be evaluated for medical causes of frequent nighttime urination. If your medical doctor finds no cause, then it's time to see urology. Everyone urinating frequently at night needs to be evaluated to be sure the bladder can empty.

FLOUROURODYNAMIC STUDIES (FUDS)

These tests are needed in the most complex incontinence cases. Many doctors have over-used them. They require well trained technicians who do the tests frequently and use standards set by the International Continence Society for the testing to be most useful. When used in the proper setting with well calibrated equipment, trained staff, and a doctor familiar with interpreting them, the testing is invaluable in diagnosing complex voiding dysfunction and complex incontinence. The best doctors to do urodynamic tests are often fellowship-trained in female urology or urogynecology. Some general urologists have developed expertise through post graduate education and extensive experience.

ELEMENTS OF THE FUDS TEST:

- Fluoroscopy is a type of low radiation X-ray used to visualize the bladder, bladder neck, urethra, and ureters.
- Cystometrogram measures how well the bladder stores and empties urine.
- Electromyography measures muscle responses from the pelvic floor. It is used to detect neuromuscular abnormalities.
- Pressure/Flow studies measure via electrodes and transducers the degree of pressure needed to void. This test diagnoses obstruction by measuring the bladder pressure required to generate a simultaneous quantified urine flow.
- Urine flow study calculates the amount of urine passed and plots the flow in milliliters per second along with the length of time needed to empty the bladder.
- A leak point pressure assessment measures how much abdominal or bladder pressure is needed for the patient to leak urine.

Entire textbooks have been written about urodynamic testing. The details are beyond our ability to describe here. Our goal is to help the patient know what to expect from the experience. You'll come to a room that might look like an operating room. Your urine will be tested to be sure you don't have an infection: if you do, the test will be cancelled. If it's normal, a very small catheter with a tiny electrode on the end will be placed into your bladder and either your vagina or rectum. These catheters will be secured to your legs.

You will sit on a toilet seat in front of an X-ray table. The nurses or technicians will fill your bladder slowly and ask you to cough, strain, and void. If the information is not obtained with the first test, your bladder might be emptied and the test repeated. You will be completely awake, as any sedatives can make the test inaccurate.

The test takes about an hour and most patients report, "it did not hurt." If your doctor is not there during the test, the results will be sent to them for interpretation and to determine the next step in your therapy. Your doctor should discuss the results at your next visit.

URETHRAL DIVERTICULUM

I'd be remiss to not mention this anatomical cause of incontinence and sometimes obstruction. The female urethra has hundreds of tiny glands that secrete mucous to help with continence by sticking the urethra tissue together. Rarely, these glands can become obstructed and dilate, which can allow urine to accumulate inside. The dilated gland or diverticulum forms a pouch and may have poor drainage and become infected. I have seen urethral diverticuli as small as a dime and as large as an orange. Your gynecologist or urologist will look for a diverticulum if you have pain in your urethra area or have leakage of urine that follows no specific pattern. Most are visualized via vaginal exam at the yearly gynecology visit.

The medical literature reports that *eight (8) percent of urethral diverticuli contain cancer*. My practice was an area referral for these surgeries, and despite performing many diverticuli removals, I only saw one case of cancer in a urethral diverticulum in 30 years. Most are asymptomatic and cause no serious harm.

I found the most common symptom to be "pain during sexual activity." I also saw diverticuli so large that they obstructed the birth process. Most patients referred to me for urethral diverticuli required surgical removal.

I mention urethral diverticuli to remind clinicians of this rare cause of incontinence and to make sure patients are evaluated for this condition prior to any other intervention.

Chapter VII

How Low Is Your T?

"Be careful about reading health books.
You may die of a misprint."

– MARK TWAIN

TESTOSTERONE REPLACEMENT IN MEN

Around 1996, I saw many men who had successful treatment for prostate cancer. By all indicators, they were *cured* of prostate cancer. But, for some, life was not worth living. CEOs of major companies, doctors, lawyers, policemen, and professors at the height of their careers were depressed, unable to focus on work, falling asleep in board meetings, and experiencing general loss of interest in life. It pained me to realize we'd cured their cancer, but taken away their desire to enjoy life.

It was fulfilling to cure the cancer, but frustrating to have an unhappy patient. I was intrigued and sought answers for my patients. I checked their thyroid. I sent many to psychiatry. I encouraged them to go to support groups. One day I decided to check their testosterone levels. I found 100% of the men who were foggy-headed, exhausted, and depressed had lower testosterone levels than expected for their age.

At this point in time, it was anathema to give supplemental testosterone to any man with prostate cancer. I talked to colleagues in endocrinology, urology, and oncology. Most had the same experience as me, but nobody was willing to treat the patients out of fear of causing the cancer to recur. When I read the world's literature on the subject, I learned that in Europe, some men had been treated with testosterone with no negative side effects. I also found that many of the men who had prostate cancer had very low testosterone levels before developing cancer. So testosterone did not seem to be the only cause of their cancer. The Endogenous Hormones and Prostate Cancer Collaborative Group published data showing, "the men with the highest risk for prostate cancer had the lowest serum testosterone."

In 1999, I began using low dose testosterone in my patients. They all knew the therapy was very controversial and I demanded they try other things first. But if the man was truly unable to function in daily life, I treated them. They had frequent follow-up visits with blood work and physical examinations. I kept their serum testosterone at levels I'd expect for a 55-year-old man, being very careful not to drive their testosterone above expected levels. The results were nothing short of amazing. My male patients were akin to a plant that needed watering and finally got a good rain. They were encouraged to exercise and follow a "Mediterranean diet," and many were sent to endocrinology to look for other causes of fatigue.

I am delighted to report that 20 years later, I never witnessed an elevation in PSA (the most common blood test for prostate cancer reoccurrence) and never had a single patient show progression of their cancer. I have heard anecdotal stories of men using testosterone for muscle growth at levels no good doctor would ever prescribe and contracting the more deadly forms of prostate cancer. I have also seen many men with metastatic prostate cancer have the disease arrested in its tracks by blocking all testosterone to their body in a lifesaving endeavor. At least since 1941, we've known castration decreased the spread of metastatic prostate cancer. When I was a surgical resident at the Veterans Affairs Medical Center in New Orleans, we did four to six castration procedures per week, with remarkable results in helping the man with metastatic prostate cancer.

I learned much in my years of giving testosterone to men. I lost many referral doctors who thought I was making a mistake, but I gained many happy patients and this many years later…it looks like I was correct. Men with specific stages of prostate cancer and low testosterone can be safely treated with very careful follow up.

Studies show testosterone may decrease fatal heart attack events, reduce body fat mass, decrease insulin resistance, increase bone density, and improve cognition. However, use of testosterone in men with known cancer remains controversial and is under ongoing study. Your urologist and oncologist who best know your case are the ones to advise you. To say that this is a complex matter is an understatement.

I will share with you what I believe from my experience. Again, this is pure opinion and your doctor should be the person advising you.

THE POWER OF ADVERTISING:

There was a 500% increase in prescriptions written for testosterone in a five-year period. This was likely due to advertisements by pharmaceutical companies and was most likely driven by patient request.

Please remember:

- Signs and symptoms of low testosterone are also symptoms of many other diseases and poor lifestyle choices.
- Low libido, poor erections, fatigue, poor sleep, foggy thinking, and loss of enthusiasm for life are common symptoms. If you have any of these problems, the first place to seek help is with your internal medicine doctor. Many conditions need to be ruled out before you consider testosterone replacement therapy.
- Before taking testosterone, remember that fat cells produce estradiol, the most potent inhibitor of testosterone production. Fat cells are loaded with aromatase that converts androgens, like testosterone, into estrogen. It is in your best interest to get to your normal body weight through diet and exercise and to attempt to build muscle before starting on a drug. Eating too much sugar and carbohydrates and drinking excessive alcohol can mimic low T.
- There are other causes of low T: opiate use, diabetes, HIV, chronic stress, sleep apnea, and steroid use. Steroids inhibit the pituitary gland from making the precursors that stimulate T production.
- Know that T levels normally decrease with age. It's called andropause. Most men and women age without needing to take hormones. Some have severe symptoms and need assistance with hormone replacement to age well.
- I observed in my own patients and saw in the literature that when men with low T were treated appropriately, their diabetes, high blood pressure, metabolic syndrome, obesity, abnormal lipid panels, and insulin resistance were more manageable. I refused to treat men unwilling to use proper diet and exercise along with T therapy.

- After your internist has ruled out all possible causes of your symptoms and your testosterone levels have been below 350 nanograms per deciliter on two blood tests drawn in the morning, (when T is naturally the highest) your doctor can try an injection of testosterone. If your symptoms are related to your low T, you will see improvement with one shot. And your symptoms will return when it wears off.

RISKS OF TAKING TESTOSTERONE:
- GYNECOMASTIA OR BREAST ENLARGMENT
- ACNE
- ERYTHROCYTOSIS OR TOO MANY RED CELLS IN YOUR BLOOD
- DECREASED SEMEN VOLUME
- INFERTILITY
- DECREASE IN TESTIS SIZE

POTENTIAL BENEFITS OF TESTOSTERONE THERAPY:
- Increased bone density and fewer fractures with aging
- Increase muscle mass
- Decreased body fat
- Increased libido and possibly sexual function
- Improved mood, sleep, and cognitive ability
- Less fatigue and depression

TREATMENT OPTIONS:
- Intramuscular injection
- Oral pill (237 mg every 12 hours)
- Transdermal patch or gel applied to the skin
- Patch applied to oral cavity every 12 hours
- Pellet implantation every three to six months

- Nasal pump

If you decide to use testosterone therapy, partner with an expert. Urologists and endocrinologists have the most education about male hormones. Be careful about using hormone clinics! Some are motivated more by profit than good medical care.

Unfortunately, I saw many patients who had been given doses of testosterone that were inappropriate for them. They felt great—right up until they had serious complications. Always check the reputation of a specialist with your primary care doctor. Internet reviews are easily manipulated and in this area cannot be trusted. Even if your primary care doctor does not support the use of testosterone therapy, they will know who to suggest you see for a second opinion.

Chapter VIII

Erectile Dysfunction is No Laughing Matter

"You only live once, but if you do it right,
once is enough."

– MAE WEST

Erectile dysfunction (ED) or impotence is the inability of a man to sustain an erection adequate for sexual activity.

The ability to enjoy sexual activity is a normal part of life. Men who can't participate are often depressed, neglect their general health, are socially isolated, and can become morose. As a urologist, it has been rewarding to help men regain function in this area.

The penis is an organ that reflects the general health of the man. It does not have a life of its own but is rather a "canary in the coal mine," particularly in younger men. If you are under 50 and having regular episodes of ED, please see your internal medicine doctor, as there is a 50% increased risk of vascular disease, heart attack, and stroke. ED may be the first symptom of vascular disease in young men.

Urologists are experts in male sexual dysfunction in the same manner that gynecologists are experts in female sexual dysfunction. Some men feel awkward talking to a woman about their ED, but my patients came specifically to discuss it with a woman. Even though it is a serious life altering condition, there was much laughter and fun in our discussions.

I had many elderly patients who were very active in retirement. One of my favorite guys was a retired airline pilot. He liked to play golf three days a week, have breakfast with his sweetie, enjoy sexual activity three days a week, and go to church on Sunday. He had a schedule he liked and it was my job to make sure "things worked properly." We were able to keep him going until the age of 86.

WHAT CAUSES AN ERECTION?

The penis is an amazing organ. Visual or tactile stimuli start a neurologic chain of events that begins in the brain. Then the muscles in the corpora cavernosa (tubes in the penis) relax and allow blood to flow in. The penis expands, closes the outflow channels, and erection is complete.

Anything affecting the man's perception, tactile input, blood flow, nerve input, or venous outflow can disturb this complex system.

WHAT CAUSES ED?
- SMOKING
- Unhealthy lifestyle
- Alcoholism and drug use
- Diabetes

- Elevated blood pressure
- Elevated cholesterol
- Obesity
- Medication
- Psychological issues
- Stress
- Atherosclerosis
- Parkinson's disease
- Multiple Sclerosis
- Sleep disorders
- Surgery of the prostate
- Spinal cord injury
- Low testosterone

As you can see from this long list, ED has many causes. The best place to start your evaluation is with your internal medicine doctor. They will rule out and treat any medical causes and refer you to urology.

EFFECTS OF STRESS ON ED

For the first 10 years I was a urologist, I almost never saw young men with ED unless they had some severe pelvic trauma (such as a fracture from car accident), a neurological condition, or severe psychological disturbance.

In the last 20 years I saw more young men with ED. The scenario was always the same. They were working 50-80 hours a week, often traveling for business, with small children at home and a partner who did not fully understand the stresses they faced. I saw the black bags under their eyes and suspected the reason for their visit: They'd fly home on Friday night, exhausted and unable to have sexual activity. The partner worried they were seeking satisfaction elsewhere, arguments ensued, performance anxiety worsened, and sexual activity became a relationship issue.

The men wanted a pill. What I gave them was counseling and stress management techniques. I'd suggest they bring their sexual partner to the next visit and we'd discuss the role of stress in ED. It's important to include your partner in this process.

I was surprised to learn that couples with young children often had sexual activity no more than once a month. These young parents spent more time at sporting events for their preschoolers than on their relationship. When I'd suggest a dinner date and adult time alone, they'd look at me like I was a lost soul. When I was a kid, the parents had their time and we had a baby sitter. I don't know when the children became the total focus of the family. But I can tell you it is not healthy for the couple's sex life!

On the other end of the spectrum is the 60-year-old obese, smoking, diabetic who can't walk easily from the couch to the refrigerator and doesn't understand why he can't get the same erections he got at 25. These men are committing slow suicide with their lifestyle choices and they want a pill or injection or surgery to keep the penis going while the rest of the body dies around it. The truth is that they are not healthy enough for sexual activity. If they did sustain a 30-minute erection, they might die from a heart attack. The only thing keeping them alive is the pharmaceutical industry and modern technology.

Getting a patient in this group to commit to changing is the most rewarding part of treating ED. It takes time to help a patient realize you are not judging them, and to become a trusted partner in their goal of rebuilding their health. Nicotine is so physically addicting that stopping smoking is harder than quitting crack cocaine. The patients find it too overwhelming to do everything at once. But often, the inability to have sexual activity is the pivotal point around choosing a healthy lifestyle.

Be prepared for a long-term project. The body did not get to this point in a few weeks and it won't get out of this condition that soon. Setting small goals with measurable results and having accountability works best. It was a big celebration in our office when a man returned having lost weight or gotten off of blood pressure or diabetes drugs. Compliments and encouragement abounded.

HOW TO DIAGNOSE ED:
- Detailed history
- Physical examination
- Blood work
- Doppler penile blood flow study, if indicated

TREATMENTS:
- Urologist working with your internist to choose medications less likely to cause ED
- Seeking psychological help when needed
- Exercise to improve blood flow to the pelvis
- Dietary changes to get to normal body weight
- Management of medical problems
- PDE-5 inhibitor medication such as Viagra,Cialis,Levitra,Stendra, (PDE-5 is an enzyme involved in the chemical pathway that controls smooth muscle activity. Blocking it allows blood to flow easily into the penis)
- Penile injection therapy
- Penile vacuum devices
- Surgery

DRUGS THAT CONTRIBUTE TO ERECTILE DYSFUNCTION ARE:
- Alcohol
- Amphetamines
- Barbiturates
- Cocaine
- Marijuana
- Methadone
- Nicotine
- Opiates

The list of prescription drugs that worsen ED is extensive and beyond the scope of our discussion. It is often difficult to determine if the disease for which the drug is prescribed is the offender or if the drug is the offender.

I strongly suggest you not stop taking any medicine prescribed by your doctor without discussion. Make sure they know of your concerns regarding ED and ask for medications less likely to worsen your problem. In some cases, your medical problems must be considered above your ED issue until you are healthy enough to make changes.

COMMON CATEGORIES OF PRESCRIPTION DRUGS THAT CAN CAUSE ED ARE:
- High blood pressure drugs
- Psychiatric medications for depression
- Anxiety medications
- Seizure medications
- Antihistamines
- Nonsteroidal anti-inflammatory drugs (NSAIDs)
- Parkinson's drugs
- Cardiac drugs

- Histamine blocking drugs
- Muscle relaxants
- Prostate cancer drugs
- Chemotherapy.

Again, please do not stop any prescribed medication without discussion with your doctor.

PSYCHOLOGICAL FACTORS IN ED

Being unable to get and keep an erection is very traumatic to most men. It is normal to occasionally have a problem with erections, commonly because of fatigue and relationship issues. After a man has difficulty, fear is often associated with sexual activity and the fear makes the problem worse.

If you get firm morning erections or erections when you are alone, there is nothing physically wrong with you. A firm morning erection implies that the arteries, veins, and nerves involved in the process are intact. If your erection troubles occur only when you are with a partner, you have a stress or psychological issue that is sometimes called performance anxiety.

The sympathetic component of our nervous system is the "fight or flight" part that controls our stress reaction. It releases compounds into the bloodstream that raise blood pressure and pulse rate. It also decreases erections. It's great if you need to run from or fight a tiger but it's not too helpful if you desire sexual activity.

My patients had success seeing certified sex therapy counsellors and using hypnotherapy, meditation, and deep breathing exercises. If the man is healthy, I prescribe three days of PDE-5 inhibitor medication to help him get and keep an erection and to build his confidence in sexual encounters. Sometimes having a few normal erections was enough to rid him of the performance anxiety.

EXERCISE

The arteries that supply the penis are connected to the arteries that supply the legs, so exercise that improves blood flow to the lower limbs can help ED. Studies in the UK have shown that walking 30 minutes per day improved erectile quality by over 50%. When I practiced in California, I saw long distance cyclists with ED, which these otherwise healthy young men induced by constant pressure on the perineum. They were treated by changing their seats, stopping the long cycle episodes, or giving up cycling altogether. If you notice numbness and tingling during cycling or afterwards, you could be pressing on the nerves to the penis and/ or temporarily decreasing the blood flow. Recreational cycling did not cause ED.

Several European studies showed Kegel exercises and work-ing with a pelvic floor physical therapist helped ED. I have no experience with this method, but imagine anything improving the muscle tone would improve the blood flow and help ED.

DIET

Several studies have shown that eating a Mediterranean or DASH (Dietary Approaches to Stop Hypertension) diet, which is more plant based as opposed to the traditional western diet with more animal protein, is associated with lower rates of ED. These studies were not "controlled" to take out exercise habits and stress factors. But if you have ED and have any medical problems, con-sider altering your diet.

MANAGEMENT OF MEDICAL PROBLEMS

Diabetes damages nerves and blood vessels that supply the penis. Clinical studies have shown that keeping blood glucose levels well controlled improves ED symptoms and can decrease chances of developing ED.

Several studies have shown improvement in ED with better management of hypertension.

Having ED is as strong a risk factor for heart disease as a history of smoking or family history of heart disease. Lowering some types of cholesterol in the blood can help prevent both heart disease and ED. All the lifestyle habits that improve your heart condition will also help with ED.

MEDICATIONS FOR ED

I remember when the FDA approved Viagra in March 1998. It had been studied for the treatment of hypertension and found to be a lousy drug for decreasing blood pressure, but was a miracle drug for ED. In six months, over five-million prescriptions were written.

The erection that would never go away was considered a possible side effect. As a young urologist, I feared my life would be ruined. I imagined men using the drug mostly on Friday and Saturday nights, and was anxiety stricken that I would spend all my weekend time in the emergency room trying to get my patients' penises out of their permanently engorged condition.

Thankfully, my worries were completely unfounded. I saw many cases of priapism due to cocaine use, spider bites, trauma, gout, sickle cell anemia, leukemia, and multiple myeloma. I never saw one case due to any PDE-5 inhibitor. Over 22 years passed from the first to the last Viagra prescription I wrote. I have been amazed at the efficacy and low side effect profile of this entire class of drugs.

TAKING NITRATES WITH PDE-5 INHIBITORS IS DANGEROUS. FATALLY LOW BLOOD PRESSURE CAN OCCUR WHEN THESE DRUGS ARE MIXED.

Since the man who has ED is also at risk for heart attack, anyone taking a PDE-5 inhibitor should make his partner aware he's using it because nitrates are commonly used in the emergency room if a heart attack is suspected. Make sure all your medications and supplements are including in your medical record. I always insisted my patients carry a complete medication list in their wallet with red stars by their ED meds in case they were taken to the ER and not able to speak. I also suggested they wear a medical alert tag, but most were unwilling to do so. I never saw a fatal low blood pressure from mixing nitrates and PDE-5 inhibitors, but my cardiology friends tell me that it can occur.

SUPPLEMENTS FOR ED

Every day men came into my office with bottles of pills they'd gotten from the internet or their alternative medicine doctor to treat ED. DHEA, L-arginine, ginseng, yohimbe, ginkgo, horny goat weed, and pomegranate were frequently compounds in these products. I never saw any of them work. The placebo effect will typically cause any drug to work more than 30% of the time but with ED, I did not observe even that effect. I did see some patients get benefit from Vitamin D, B3 (niacin), and folic acid if their diet was deficient or their blood levels low. It may be that the patients who came to see me had tried supplements that failed. There could be some folks who got better with supplements and never sought medical care.

Yohimbe is a supplement I consider unsafe. It causes elevated blood pressure and irregular heart rhythm. I advise against trying it. Even though I like the name *horny goat weed,* I also advise against its use as I have seen it cause cardiac arrhythmias and low blood pressure.

HORMONES

I read article after article claiming there is no relationship between testosterone and erectile dysfunction. They claimed that testosterone was necessary for desire. But in the man with normal desire and poor erections, it was reported as not helpful in every study I read. In point of fact, in 2022 when you search Google, the results still say testosterone won't help the quality of erections.

That is NOT my clinical experience. Ninety percent of my patients using testosterone supplementation for serum levels of low T reported improvement in erections. Keep in mind that I insisted these men exercise, watch their diet, and lose weight if they were obese. Their medical care had multiple factors. When changing more than one variable at a time, it is impossible to determine which change caused the effect. Most of my patients' partners did notice a decrease in erectile quality at the end of the dosing interval in patients using injections or pellets for administration of their medicine.

ERECTION CONSTRICTION TENSION RINGS

If you get an erection but the blood flow seems to seep out before you can complete activity, a carefully placed ring around the base of the penis can decrease the venous outflow and solve your problem. The International Society for Sexual Medicine describes on their website how to safely use a penile ring. Be sure you remove it as soon as activity is over. I have gone to the emergency room to remove a few in my career.

Penile rings are most comfortable when the hair at the base of the penis is shaved and lubrication is used. Some patients purchased them on Amazon. My suggestion is to be gentle with your penis and remove the ring right after activity. If you are on a blood thinner, impressive bruising can occur.

PENILE VACUUM CONSTRICTION DEVICES

When I was a resident studying urology at five different Veterans Affairs Medical Centers, around the country, the FDA approved these devices and our veterans were able to get them with a prescription. They work by pulling blood into the penis externally and using a constricting band at the base of the penis to keep the blood in during activity.

I was surprised that 75% of the men using the device were happy with it as a treatment for ED. However, this was before the days of PDE-5 inhibitors. In my later clinical practice, the combination of the pill and the vacuum device was popular with men in stable, one-partner relationships. It proved too cumbersome in short- term scenarios.

PENILE INJECTION THERAPY

In this mode of therapy, the patient or his partner is taught to give an injection directly into the penis five to 15 minutes prior to desired activity. The therapy uses multiple compounded agents. I found alprostadil, phentolamine, prostaglandin E1, and papaverine worked best. Your urologist will help choose the best agent for you.

The drugs increase blood flow into the penis by relaxing the smooth muscle and widening the blood vessels. Many men were frightened at the thought of injecting their penis with a tiny needle, but when the patient had an open mind and was properly trained, excellent results occurred. Complications of bruising, priapism and Peyronie's plaques were extremely rare. I think our low complication rate was due to intense instruction, clear communication, and choosing the right patient for the therapy.

In the last few years, *men's sexual treatment clinics* have popped up. I have no inside knowledge of what goes on in these places. I did see many men in the emergency room for relief of priapism after they had been given the highest doses of medication for penile injection. I suggest you talk to your urologist before going to one of these clinics. The lowest dose of drug that gives an adequate erection is the best approach. As with any medication, do not use more than is needed.

SURGERY

I stopped doing penile implant surgery for erectile dysfunction in the late 1990's. There were frequent device failures and the patients often had unrealistic expectations. Those with diabetes sometimes got infections. Many thought the device would enlarge their penises, which it does not. Some had numbness at the surgical site.

If you have tried all options and surgery is the only one left, go to a urologist who does this operation all the time. Many men have been helped and had excellent surgical outcomes in the hands of urologic surgeons who perform the procedures frequently. It is my understanding that the devices used today fail far less often than the models I used in the early 90's. However, surgery should still be the last resort.

EXTRACORPOREAL SHOCK WAVE LITHOTRIPSY (ESWL) TO THE PENIS FOR ED

There are clinics offering treatments to "stimulate penile tissue" and encourage blood flow, and claiming that, "low intensity shock waves improve blood flow to the penis." I have no experience with this mode of therapy being successful. Six of my patients went to a clinic and spent $6,000 each trying this therapy and returned to report that it didn't work.

New technology comes out every year. Before spending a lot of money on anything, I'd suggest you get the details and discuss it with your urologist. There may be excellent treatments not listed in my chapter. But don't fall for a savvy sales pitch without consulting your urologist. I have seen impressive websites and great testimonials for treatments that do not work and are sometimes harmful.

Chapter IX

The Kidney Stone
Always Wins!

"I will not cut, even for the stone, but I will leave such procedures to the practitioners of that craft."
– HIPPOCRATIC OATH (GREEK TEXT 275 AD)

The earliest reported kidney stone was found in a mummy in Egypt dated around 4800 BC. One in ten people will form a stone in their lifetime.

When I'm called to the emergency room to see a patient with a kidney stone, I don't have to ask which person is my patient. It's an easy diagnosis to make from the hallway. The unlucky person writhing in pain, looking wild-eyed and desperate for any treatment to relieve their agony is the one. I work in a hospital that has one of the busiest obstetrics wards in the southeast. My patients who have had natural childbirth and passed kidney stones report, "they'd rather have a baby every day than have another kidney stone." I don't know why passing kidney stones is hideously painful but I have seen many patients made crazy by the pain.

After operating on others for 30 years, I had first-hand experience with a kidney stone. I never want another. My husband and I, perpetually ten pounds overweight, decided to try the Keto diet after a friend lost 22 pounds on it in three months, which sounded appealing. We studied the diet and began our high-protein adventure. Many good things happened. My recalcitrant psoriasis was gone in two weeks. We had more energy and the weight fell off for the first month. All was well, for a while.

At my age, height, and sex, I should eat approximately 56 grams of protein per 24 hours. When on the Keto diet, I ingested more than 100 grams in that time.

One afternoon, when I was walking down the hall to see one of my favorite patients, I got a jolt of severe pain in my left lower abdomen. It felt like I'd imagine being tasered would feel. I had never felt any such pain in my life.

I paused in the hall, took a deep breath, and thought *that was a heck of a bowel spasm*. I continued my work, urinated two hours later, and found the toilet in my office full of my own bloody urine. It had never occurred to me I might have a kidney stone. I guzzled water, tried not to panic, and finished seeing the afternoon's patients.

I felt normal until two in the morning when I awoke with pain that I thought might kill me. I don't have pain medicine at home and decided to try to tough it out. For two hours, I cried like a baby, rocking and flailing on my toilet, and thrashing around on the bathroom floor. I threw up and fought to not faint.

Around four a.m., a tiny black stone smaller than a BB popped out of my urethra onto the toilet paper. My first words were, "You little bastard! That's it? I thought I was giving birth to a boulder!"

How could something that tiny cause such agony? I'd listened to patients describe this phenomenon. I had taken thousands to the operating room to relieve their misery. But there is nothing like first-hand experience. I now know why the kidney stone patient looks deranged. I know the terror of a toilet full of blood. I understand why the patients stand in front of the triage nurse in the emergency room and beg for pain medication. Passing a kidney stone is horrendous!

Diet is important in the prevention of stones. NO MORE VERY HIGH PROTIEN DIET FOR ME!

HOW TO DECREASE KIDNEY STONE FORMATION:
- Drink enough fluid to make between 2.5 and three liters of urine per 24 hours.
- Avoid alcohol, caffeine, sugar, and sodium containing beverages.
- Lemon water is likely the best beverage for stone formers.
- Avoid sodium in the diet (less than 2300 mg. per 24 hours).
- Most people do not need to limit calcium.
- The best diet is the DASH diet.
- Unless you are one of the very rare hyperoxaluria patients, fruits and vegetables are your friends. Primary hyperoxaluria is an inherited disease in which the liver doesn't produce enough of an enzyme that prevents the over production of oxalate. The excess ends up in the kidneys and forms stones.
- Avoid vitamin C.
- Eat no more than 0.7 grams/kg. /day of protein.
- Take Theralith XR.
- Consider taking potassium citrate, hydrochlorothiazide or chlorthaladone if your 24-hour urine demonstrates the prescription drugs to be efficacious.

HOW DO THESE SUGGESTIONS WORK?

Kidney stones are formed from crystals. Remember the crystal garden experiment most of us did in school where you put anions (negatively charged particles) and cations (positively charged particles) together in water and VOILA...crystals grow? Kidney stone formation is similar. Given the right set of circumstances, almost anyone can form a stone.

Most people don't make kidney stones because our ingenious bodies adapted over many years to handle the Western diet. Carnivores and omnivores rid the vast amount of acidic food we eat through beautiful and complex mechanisms in the gut, the kidneys, and our bones. What happens in our kidneys is much more complicated, but similar to the crystal experiment.

DRINK THE RIGHT AMOUNT OF FLUIDS

Sufficient fluid intake keeps the components of the crystals in solution. If the urine is concentrated, meaning you have not had much to drink, the components of the crystals can "find" one another more easily. If one grain of salt is dissolved in one gallon of water, the two parts, sodium, and chloride, will have a hard time finding each other to "stick back together." If the two grains of salt are in one half cup of water, they might find it easy to reconvene and form a crystal.

I apologize to the physical chemists for my simplistic explanation. I suspect drinking lots of fluid flushes the crystals out by diluting the urine, decreasing urine acidity, removing excess salt, and keeping the urine going in one direction... out the toilet.

In summary: water flushes crystals out and keeps them from sticking together in solution.

AVOID SODIUM IN YOUR DIET

Excess sodium in the diet contributes to many problems. It raises the blood pressure and leads to heart disease. It is nearly impossible to frequently dine out and maintain a normal sodium intake. Watch professional chefs grab a bowl of salt and toss handfuls into the food. It's a great flavor enhancer but is unhealthy for most people.

When my husband and I eat at home in a healthy manner, and then go to one of our favorite restaurants for dinner, the next day I cannot wear my rings, my shoes are tight, and I have gained a pound of fluid.

Ingesting salt causes calcium to be released into the kidneys. Chronically eating more sodium than needed can lead to osteoporosis and kidney stones. Sodium exits the kidney attached to calcium. For years I've reviewed patients' 24-hour urine collections and when I see elevated calcium, I almost always see elevated urine sodium. So even if my patient thinks they are eating low sodium, the 24-hour urine tells the true tale. For most people, 1500–2300 mg of sodium per 24 hours is normal consumption. Reading food labels is the only way to learn to eat properly for kidney stone prevention.

In a diet chronically high in sodium intake, calcium reabsorption (calcium taken back into the body from the urine) is decreased and the calcium ends up in the urine. One of the fastest ways to make a calcium oxalate kidney stone is to eat a high sodium diet with high animal protein. In retrospect, I wish I had given my business cards out at the local steak houses…particularly the ones with the greater than eight-ounce steaks!

MOST PEOPLE DO NOT NEED TO LIMIT CALCIUM

Unless you are consuming large volumes of calcium-containing foods, you don't need to limit calcium. In fact, studies have shown that people who did severely limit calcium intake were more likely to make stones.

If you are a calcium oxalate stone former, it might be best to eat your high oxalate foods along with your high calcium foods. For example, have your spinach salad with a glass of milk. The oxalate and calcium bind together in your gut and whatever your body does not need goes out in your stool and not your urine. This is a simplistic explanation for a complex process, but it is easy to comprehend.

Whatever you take in that your body does not need is processed in a few ways.

You exhale, urinate, sweat and defecate excesses, and sometimes your body chooses to store things for later. Usually if we give the body what it needs, it will take care of the rest. Sometimes we overwhelm the body and disease results.

What about calcium supplements? I am not an expert in osteoporosis and quite frankly, the literature on osteoporosis is confusing even to doctors. But if your physician advises you to take a calcium supplement and you are a stone former, the best way to take the supplement is to use 500 mg. of calcium citrate after your largest meal of the day and chase it with 10 oz. of lemon water. There is NO scientific proof that this always works in everyone, but over many years, I have not seen stone formation increase in people who follow this advice. If you have osteoporosis and form calcium oxalate stones, you might benefit from seeing a nephrologist who focuses on kidney stone prevention.

As the famous stone guru, Dr. Fredric L. Coe once said, "A low calcium diet is bad for anyone with a skeleton."

TRY THE DASH DIET (DIETARY APPROACHES TO STOP HYPERTENSION)

Many discoveries in medicine are found by accident. The DASH diet was designed to lower blood pressure and decrease heart attack and stroke risk. But when kidney stone formers were included in a study, the incidence of stone formation went down dramatically. Some kidney stones are more likely to form in an acid environment. The DASH diet helps to create an alkaline environment in which the stones are less likely.

DRINK CITRUS BEVERAGES

Several studies have shown drinking lemon water or eating oranges can reduce the incidence of kidney stones. The most common prescription drug used to prevent stones is potassium citrate. The citrate component is thought to increase urine pH or alkalize the urine, while helping to prevent stone particles from sticking together and growing.

This may also be how lemon water helps. One popular recipe for lemon water is to put one cup of fresh lemon juice in eight cups of spring water and drink it every day. Be sure to rinse your mouth afterward as the lemon can erode tooth enamel. Some people with GERD (gastroesophageal reflux disease) cannot tolerate lemon. I suggest my patients do the best they can with the citrus ingestion. The water consumption is most likely the most important component of stone prevention, and some researchers don't believe citrus intake matters.

EAT FRUITS AND VEGETABLES

The more fruits and vegetables you eat, the better. In rare cases this is incorrect. If you have the rare condition of primary hyperoxaluria, you may have to eat a low oxalate diet. However, the only way to know if you fit into that group is if you have had blood work and a 24 hour-urine evaluation. I can count on one hand the number of pure primary hyperoxaluria patients I've ever seen.

The more fruits and vegetables you consume, the more alkaline your urine will be, and the less likely you are to form the most common types of stones.

VITAMIN C

Every decade I've been a doctor I've seen the "wonder vitamin of the decade," including Vitamin E, Zinc, Vitamin B-12, Vitamin D, and Vitamin C. Each has benefits and each has toxicity. Vitamin C can increase urinary oxalates and I prefer that stone patients not take too much. By all means, get it in food but don't take extra. In the winter I see patients taking unbelievable amounts of Vitamin C because they believe it wards off colds and flu. If you must take vitamin C, please do not take more than 1000 mg per day. If you know you form calcium oxalate kidney stones, get vitamin C in food.

One of my favorite patients, who is a stone former and whose father is a stone former, called me distraught over her four-year-old daughter. She said, "I have taken my daughter to three doctors for urinary frequency and urgency. She is suffering with her bladder. I know you don't see children, but we are desperate. She has been checked for infection and all is negative. She urinates every twenty minutes around the clock and holds her privates and cries, "Mommy, it hurts."

I saw the child and sat with her mother to inquire about her diet. She had been giving the child Vitamin C to ward off the flu, so the child was forming calcium oxalate crystals and the crystals were irritating her bladder. She stopped all vitamin C and the child was "cured" of her bladder issues. Her story is a wonderful example of two principles: Too much of a good thing is too much, and just because it is "natural" doesn't mean it can't harm you.

PROTEIN

Fredric Coe, M.D. also said, "Like all dietary factors in stone disease, protein is complex."

Excess animal protein found in eggs, red meat, poultry, and seafood can increase the amount of uric acid in the urine. A high protein diet can also lower the urinary production of citrate, an important chemical in stone prevention. High protein diets can reduce the body's ability to absorb calcium and increase its acid load, which causes excretion of calcium in the urine. Ingesting animal protein also boosts the excretion of oxalate, and chronic high protein diets cause bone loss by the excretion of calcium.

Common sense dictates: If an acid load causes you to lose calcium and an alkali load causes you to lose less calcium, would long-term chronic acidosis cause you to lose bone? Most likely it would. But one thing is certain: all the studies show acidic urine has high urinary calcium and more alkaline urine has less calcium. Whether this translates into diet preventing bone loss or not, I don't know. But excess calcium in the urine most certainly leads to kidney stones.

If you are a calcium oxalate kidney stone former, I suggest you adhere to the following:

- If you are a female, eat 0.7 grams of protein per kilogram of body weight per 24 hours.
- If you are a male, you can have as much as one gram of protein per kilo of body weight every 24 hours.

To calculate an individual's proper protein intake for a 24-hour period:

- First determine your weight in kilograms by multiplying your weight in pounds by 0.454. For example: 200 pounds x 0.454 = 90.8 kilograms.
- If you are a 200-pound man, one gram of protein per kilogram of body weight = 90.8 grams of protein per 24 hours.
- If you are a female and weigh 150 pounds: 150 pounds x 0.454 = 68.1 kilograms X 0.7 grams = 47.67 grams of protein per 24 hours.

There are approximately 50 grams of protein in a lean eight-ounce steak. One egg has approximately six grams of protein. Most protein powders have about 20 grams of protein per scoop.

THERALITH XR

TheraLith XR is a nutritional supplement for prevention of kidney stones. It contains magnesium, potassium, and vitamin B6, all of which block stone formation. It is available with an extended-release coating to decrease stomach upset.

Prescription strength potassium citrate causes stomach upset in some patients. Often insurance plans only pay for the generic form of the drug, which many patients can take with no upset but some are unable to tolerate. Some patients report diarrhea on potassium citrate. I can't explain why, but most folks don't have the upset with the branded form of the drug (Urocit-K). I suspect there is a difference in the delivery system.

Because potassium citrate is not well tolerated by every patient, I was excited when a quality supplement was created to decrease stone formation and have fewer side effects. Studies show TheraLith XR increases urinary magnesium and citrate (both stone blockers) and decreases calcium oxalate crystals. The product is gluten free. Two pills every 12 hours after a meal is my suggestion.

If you can tolerate and afford prescription strength potassium citrate, it may be more efficacious in repetitive calcium oxalate stone formers. I have not found a study comparing the two, but I have seen great results with both products.

If you do not have normal kidney function, please check with your doctor before taking any supplement and always include all supplements with your drug list at every visit.

PRESCRIPTION DRUGS TO PREVENT STONES
HOW DOES POTASSIUM CITRATE HELP?

Potassium is an element, a metal on the periodic table. The body needs it to support many functions. The recommended daily dose of potassium from food is 3500–4700 mg. per 24 hours. Beets, white beans, soy beans, and lima beans are potassium-rich foods. My favorite high-potassium foods are avocados, spinach, sweet potatoes, and broccoli.

Citrate is an organic compound, $C_6H_8O_7$, that occurs naturally in citrus fruits. It inhibits calcium oxalate and calcium phosphate precipitation. Remember that citric acid can erode tooth enamel and rinse your mouth liberally after ingesting citrus fruit.

Potassium citrate attaches to the calcium in the urine and prevents the calcium from attaching to other things that can form crystals, which are the building blocks of stones. The drug alkalizes the urine to help prevent stones. Many researchers consider a urine pH between 6.0 and 7.0 to be ideal to prevent stones. If your urine pH is persistently higher or lower, you might be at increased risk for stone formation, if you are predisposed. Citrate alone inhibits crystal formation.

Citrate occurs naturally in the body and has important roles. If you eat a diet high in acid, the diet alone will deliver less citrate to your kidneys. If you eat a diet high in fruits and vegetables, your system will be more alkaline and deliver more citrate to your urine. The higher the citrate, the less likely you are to make stones. If you are disciplined about reducing protein in the diet, especially animal protein, and diligent in increasing all types of fruits and vegetables, you might avoid taking potassium citrate.

What does potassium (K+) have to do with all of this? Depletion of potassium in the body lowers the pH in the kidney cells and lowers urinary citrate.

Potassium citrate in doses of 10-30 mg every eight hours neutralizes a large fraction of dietary acid. Your physician will check your blood work to be sure this medication is safe for you.

HCTZ (HYDROCHLOROTHIAZIDE) AND CHLORTHALIDONE AND INDAPAMIDE

This category of drugs is known as the thiazide diuretics. When used at therapeutic doses, they decrease calcium stone formation. There are a dozen studies in the medical literature comparing calcium stone formers who took no thiazide diuretic to those that did. While the group of patients receiving no drug had a 50% chance of making another stone, the group on thiazides had a 75% chance of NOT making a new stone.

Many experts in stone physiology believe the combination of a thiazide diuretic and potassium citrate works best for calcium stone formers. My personal experience has been that without diet and lifestyle changes, patients continue to make stones. The same patient who won't drink fluids and avoid sodium may be the one who also forgets to take their medication. Poor compliance causes any prevention program to fail.

How do the drugs work? Some patients think they increase urine output and can substitute for drinking lots of fluid. That may be true for the first few days, but the body will equalize itself quickly, and what comes in will go out.

If you don't have adequate fluid intake, a diuretic will eventually cause dehydration, which is the enemy of the stone former. Thiazides are NOT a substitute for fluid intake. These drugs lower urinary calcium and ph. Thiazide diuretics help put calcium back into the bones, which is one reason they have been a favorite treatment for older patients with bone loss.

Thiazides can deplete potassium which can decrease urinary citrate, and both can increase stone formation. Patients taking thiazides need a high potassium diet or should take potassium citrate.

Thiazides remove sodium from the body and can lower blood pressure. But if the patient ingests too much sodium, the diet can override the sodium wasting effect. Don't think you can eat whatever you want and take these drugs. Diet and medication are the order of the day. Loss of potassium is made worse by a diet high in sodium. Your doctor will check your blood work to be sure the electrolyte balance is favorable.

BEST DOSES FOR CALCIUM OXALATE STONE FORMERS:
- Chlorthalidone 12.5 mg per day (half of a 25 mg pill)
- Indapamide 1.25 mg per day
- Hydrochlorothiazide 12.5 mg every 12 hours

INFECTION STONES

I worked with many obese diabetic patients with infection stones. The stones are composed of struvite and will not resolve without adequate treatment of the infection. Some bacteria produce ammonia that makes the urine alkaline. If the urine becomes too alkaline, these stones form.

If your doctor finds urine infections with the same organism repetitively, or if you pass stones composed of magnesium ammonium phosphate or calcium carbon-apatite, be sure your urologist is aware. In my practice, struvite stones were the largest I saw. Most needed percutaneous nephrolithotomy, which is minimally invasive surgery that involves making a hole in the back to break and extract the stone in pieces. They can be difficult to manage as the infection can be hard to clear.

WHAT ABOUT TOPAMAX (TOPIRAMATE)?

Topamax is a drug used to treat migraines and other types of chronic pain. It can cause renal tubular acidosis where the kidneys cannot process acid properly and patients form calcium phosphate stones. Unfortunately, taking a thiazide diuretic and potassium citrate will not combat the propensity to make stones on Topamax, in my experience.

If you are a stone former and must take Topamax for another medical reason, I suggest you see a nephrologist specializing in stone prevention to assist with this complex problem. I have not seen stone formers successfully take Topamax.

HOW DO WE DIAGNOSE YOUR INDIVIDUAL CAUSE OF STONE FORMATION?

- If you pass a stone, dry it off and take it to your urologist. We send it to a lab that knows within a week what kind of stone it is. Unfortunately, some people have been known to pass more than one type.
- We use 24-hour urine collection compared with blood work to analyze factors in your blood and urine that lead to stone formation. Your doctor will look for a rare disease called hyperparathyroidism that can disturb your body's

handling of calcium and will check for gout and dietary indiscretions. Unless otherwise instructed, it's best to stop all supplements during collection of the urine and to eat and drink as you normally would to help your doctor get the most accurate information.

- Be sure to give your doctor detailed information about your family if you have stone formers. Knowing what kind of stones your family members make can be helpful.

Chapter X

Kidney Stone Surgery

"We will either find a way or make one."

– HANNIBAL (247 BC)

When I was a budding young urologist, we often did open kidney stone surgery. Occasionally, the patient had a stone in the perfect place for a small back incision, but complex surgery required cutting the body almost in half. The patient was incised from the belly button around to their mid-back and the kidney was cut open to remove the larger stones.

It was exciting from the standpoint of the surgeon and was one of the procedures that drew me to the field of urology. From the patient's perspective, it was hideous. The postoperative pain was grueling and the recovery took eight to 12 weeks. Long hospitalizations were not uncommon. Most folks were out of work for at least four to six weeks. And there were complications. Because the kidneys are adjacent to the lower lungs, some patients developed pneumonia because they could not take deep breaths due to pain.

Writings about bladder stones being removed through the perineum have been dated as far back as 40 AD. Articles about surgery to remove kidney stones began appearing in the late 1800s. From about 1875 until 1985, there was little progress in technique. But urology has always been in the forefront of new technology. We love our gadgets.

By the time I'd finished my years in general surgery, we very infrequently performed open stone surgery. By the time I became a chief resident, I never saw another open stone surgery case. From 1985 to 1990 our field advanced so fast that it became rare to make a traditional incision for kidney stone removal.

Patients ask about *dissolving their stones.* Uric acid stones are caused by high levels of uric acid in your blood. Pure uric acid stones form in urine with a pH below 5.5, while the rare cystine stones (less than one percent of all stones) form at pH below 6.5. If the urine was constantly held at a pH above this number and the stones were pure, they could be dissolved. I have never successfully *dissolved* a pure Cystine stone.

RISK FACTORS FOR URIC ACID STONES:
- Obesity
- History of chemotherapy
- Diabetes
- Diet high in salt and sugar
- Diet high in animal protein
- Family history of uric acid stones
- Gout

Fifteen percent of the stones I saw were uric acid stones. Most in my practice were mixed with calcium oxalate and were not amenable to dissolving. But if you pass pure uric acid stones, potassium citrate could help alkalize your urine and decrease the stone burden. I had universally poor results dissolving stones because the metabolic and dietary issues causing their formation continued to exist.

Today we use:

- ESWL, extracorporeal shock wave lithotripsy. The patient's stone is located using radiology techniques and shock waves are passed through the body until the stone is broken. The patient passes the smaller fragments later.

- Ureteroscopy with holmium laser lithotripsy and basket stone extraction is the most common procedure for stones in the ureter, the tube from the kidney to the bladder. With the patient under anesthesia, we pass a small fiber optic scope through the urethra and up to the stone and apply holmium laser energy to break it. Large fragments are trapped in a basket and brought down the ureter and out the body. Sometimes, a small stent is left to help drain the kidney afterwards. The technology evolves yearly. The brilliant engineers who design these technologies are always working to make the scopes smaller and the lasers more accurate.

- Percutaneous nephrolithotomy is used for large stones in the center or pelvis of the kidney. The procedure involves making small holes in the back and kidney and working through a port to break and remove stones. This procedure is more invasive and less frequently used than the first two, but it works better under specific conditions. Your urologist will know when to use it.

- Robotic removal is used for large stones in the kidney also. The position of the stone will determine which approach works best.

- Removing a kidney for stone disease is rare. It is used only in cases where the stones are so large that they have chronically obstructed and damaged the kidney such that removal (or nephrectomy) is the only answer.

Unfortunately, our great technology has not led to decreased formation of stones. What we have exchanged from the patient's standpoint is: greatly decreased pain with no need to be out of work for months at a time in return for the potential of multiple minor procedures.

When we opened patients' kidneys we could easily get all the particles out. Now, particularly with ESWL, we know fragments are left behind that likely require subsequent, less invasive surgery. To reiterate, we've exchanged one very invasive procedure with serious complications for multiple less invasive procedures with fewer complications.

Chapter XI

Prostate Cancer

Prostate Cancer– *PRIMUM, NON NOCERE* (First, do no harm)

*"It's not enough to be busy, so are the ants.
The question is, what are we busy about?"*
– HENRY DAVID THOREAU

Many books have been written to educate patients about prostate cancer (CAP). Most major medical centers have excellent websites with much information about the disease. My goal is to give the man and his partner the information they need to develop questions prior to their doctors' visits, because it is a complex topic.

WHAT IS THE PROSTATE?

When normal, it is a small gland between the neck of your bladder and the sphincter that you relax to urinate. For most of the time I was a urologist we did not know what it did. We now know it produces fluid to nourish sperm.

Prostate cancer is fascinating in that it has at least two forms. One type causes almost no trouble to the patient. A man can live his life and never know he has it. Another form is deadly. It's aggressive, grows fast, and will end your life and make you quite miserable in the process.

The doctor's dilemma is in trying to figure out who to screen, who to diagnose, and who to treat. And all of these questions are complicated.

During my 33 years as a practicing urologist, I tended to be aggressive in diagnosing and treating prostate cancer. My view was skewed and biased because of the men I saw die hideous deaths from prostate cancer. I'll never forget the first patient I ever saw with CAP. He was an attractive African American man 52 years of age. He and his wife were in the emergency room because he had had right lower abdominal pain which they thought was appendicitis.

As the surgery resident on call, I went to evaluate him and report to my faculty surgeon. His entire abdomen was rock hard. He had lost weight without dieting over the last three months and had severe back pain. He did not have appendicitis; he had prostate cancer, the aggressive form. It had spread throughout his abdomen, had caused a bowel obstruction, and had widely metastasized to his bones. Despite having an orchiectomy to remove his testes as a source of testosterone stimulation to the tumor, and aggressive radiation therapy, he died within four months. I'll never forget him. He fought bravely. He was otherwise quite healthy and had not been to a doctor in ten years. His wife recalled that in his family history, "Several men had died of cancer, but they did not know what type."

Thankfully, this has been a rare scenario since the advent of the PSA screening test. PSA, prostate specific antigen, is a cancer marker first discovered around 1960 and FDA-approved to aid in diagnosing prostate cancer in 1986.

Prostate cancer has no specific common symptoms until it has spread. It's a bit like ovarian cancer in that respect. You don't know you have it until it's nearly too late to cure it. Unlike other cancers, some prostate cancer does not need treatment. In fact, in some cases, "the treatment is worse than the problem." The work of the clinician is in trying to figure out who should be screened and who should be treated, and what treatment is appropriate.

FACTORS THAT INCREASE RISK:
- Men related to you by blood with CAP
- Being of African descent (African American), as the cancer is often more aggressive in men of African descent
- Family history of breast cancer with BRCA-1 or BRCA-2
- Strong family history of any form of breast cancer
- Being over 50
- Obesity

What causes CAP? We do not know. All cancers come from changes in the DNA of the affected cells. Abnormal instructions occur at the gene level and some cells take over and grow abnormally. Prostate cancer can spread locally, and it can metastasize into the blood and go to distant organs.

My goal is to help you think about prostate cancer from the patient's perspective. The first question is should you get screened or not? Prostate cancer has no symptoms in the early stages. The screening tests are: 1) Digital rectal exam (DRE) and 2) blood testing with PSA or other cancer markers. Both are imperfect. Neither can tell you if you have cancer or not. If both are totally normal, you can worry less. If either is abnormal, it requires follow-up and often biopsy.

Over the last decade, several medical groups have suggested that your primary care doctor not do DRE and not order prostate cancer screening blood work. They have suggested that prostate cancer has been "over treated by urologists." There is some merit to their concerns. But since there are no signs or symptoms of prostate cancer until the disease has progressed, is it best to do no screening?

As a patient, I would not want that approach. I prefer to be informed about the pros and cons of screening and allowed to make my own personal decision. If I'm at risk, and I'm in otherwise good health, I want to be screened. If I'm in very poor health and could not undergo treatment safely, I might not want to be screened. The danger of choosing to not be screened is that you have a treatable disease and miss the window of opportunity for cure. The danger of choosing to be screened is that you undergo needless testing with the loss of time and money in pursuit of problems that don't exist. It's a tough choice for the doctor and the patient.

The important thing about prostate cancer screening is that the patient knows what they are choosing and trusts their doctor to guide them. Since prostate cancer is so complex, I'd suggest you see a urologist if you have men with prostate cancer in your family or if you are African American and over 50. Remember that you don't have to do anything just because the doctor recommends it. If you are not totally comfortable with your options, another opinion from an expert is always a good idea.

Since we don't know what causes prostate cancer, we can't offer in-depth suggestions for prevention. But we do know a few things that correlate with lower risks of most cancers:

- Eat lots of fresh, colorful fruits and vegetables. They appear to contain antioxidants that have cancer protective effects.
- Exercise most days. Studies suggest 150 minutes per week.
- Maintain close to your ideal body weight.
- Don't rely on supplements. None have proven to decrease the incidence of CAP.
- The jury is still out on the use of 5 alpha reductase inhibitor (finasteride, dutasteride) prescription drugs for prostate cancer prevention. There are studies that show these drugs decrease the chance of getting CAP and other studies that show long-term use of this drug class may be associated with developing the most aggressive forms of CAP. Discuss this topic with your urologist to get the most up to date information.

IF YOU DECIDE PROSTATE CANCER SCREENING IS RIGHT FOR YOU, WHAT SHOULD YOU EXPECT?

- DRE – digital rectal examination.
- Blood test – PSA. There are other cancer screening tests that are less commonly used. Your urologist will know the latest information in the urologic literature. Follow their suggestions.
- Possible MRI of the prostate. This tool is excellent in the hands of a radiologist trained in prostate MRI, with a dedicated prostate MRI machine, and a technician who does the procedure frequently. It is a specialized high-tech test that is under scrutiny. New studies are coming out all the time to help the urologist know where this technology is best used. It's expensive but could save the patient an invasive prostate biopsy.

- Possible ultrasound guided prostate biopsy. Prostate biopsy with the Gleason's score for cancer is the current gold standard. The biopsy can miss cancer because it is not taking out the entire gland, only sampling it. When MRI guidance is added to prostate biopsy, the accuracy goes up, but so does the cost.

If you choose to have a prostate biopsy, you'll get a Gleason's score from the pathologist looking at your tissue. The Gleason's score is very important. A book could easily be written about the score and its use in CAP. A very simplistic way to think about it is that the higher the score, the more trouble the CAP can cause the patient. A Gleason's score can be anywhere from 2-10.

GLEASON'S SCORE IN GENERAL:
- Less than 6 is considered low grade CAP
- 7 is medium grade CAP
- Over 8 is high grade CAP

Sometimes your urologist will order genomic testing to help give you a more accurate prognosis. Genomic testing is not always needed. Please remember my explanations are very simplistic. I am hoping to provide a framework upon which you can begin to work out questions for your urologist.

CURRENT TREATMENTS FOR CAP:
- Active surveillance. If your PSA is in the low range and your Gleason's score from your prostate biopsy is low, you may be considered for active surveillance. It involves having regular DRE and blood testing and occasional repeat

prostate biopsy. Most men do not progress to need further treatment, but some do.

- Surgery – Perineal or abdominal or robot-assisted laparoscopic prostatectomy (prostate removal). This is major surgery, but the techniques are excellent and most patients either go home the same day or within 24 – 36 hours. Be sure you go to a urologist who does this procedure every week.
- External beam radiation therapy. Radiation is sent from an external source through your body to the affected area (prostate and tissue around the prostate and sometimes to bone metastasis).
- Proton beam therapy is a form of radiation therapy. The centers doing it claim it delivers a more focused energy to the affected organ with less local tissue damage. I am not certain this is true in all cases. Talk to your urologist before showing up at one of these facilities for care.
- Brachytherapy, in which tiny seeds are implanted in your prostate gland to radiate it from the inside out. It is most often an outpatient procedure.
- Cryoablation – Freezing abnormal prostate tissue.
- HIFU – High Intensity Focused Ultrasound or heating the abnormal prostate tissue.
- Orchiectomy is the removal of the testicles. In metastatic hormone-sensitive CAP this treatment works very well. It is used most often in the elderly male with severe cancer and poor general health.
- Drugs – there are multiple drugs that decrease testosterone or block testosterone. Your urologist will guide you to the right one.
- Chemotherapy.
- Immunotherapy.

- There are currently no known alternative therapies that predictably kill CAP.

Prostate cancer is complex. A patient can have a normal PSA and have cancer, or have an abnormal PSA and not have cancer. A patient also can have a normal biopsy and have cancer. My advice is to read this information and write your questions as you go. If you want to read about prostate cancer, go to the websites for major centers like the Mayo Clinic, the Cleveland Clinic, MD Anderson, and WebMD. There are hundreds of patient-oriented books, some of them quackery. Dr. Andrew Siegel's book *Prostate Cancer 20/20* has a balanced approach with information that was accurate up to 2019.

When approaching this topic, remember that whomever you visit feels that what they do is the best treatment. It's human nature. If someone spent many years improving their talent at a particular task, they have to believe it works. The HIFU guy will think HIFU is the best. The proton beam guy thinks his treatment is best. The robotic guy is sure his surgery is the best. None of these doctors have any ill intent. They will have the prejudice that their technique is the best technique. The best doctors will give you options and explain why some are suited for you.

If you are diagnosed with prostate cancer, take someone with you to the visit and expect the doctor to spend time with you. This is not a fifteen-minute discussion. Do not rush yourself. Take time to listen, take notes, write questions. and consider other opinions. Do NOT go to ten people to get their opinions because you'll drive yourself crazy. But know that there are gray areas in treating prostate cancer and there is no one best option for everyone.

On a positive note…prostate cancer is more treatable and curable than ever before. In the last 25 years, I have not seen a patient in the dire straits that my first prostate cancer patient faced. We are diagnosing the disease earlier, treating it smarter, and our techniques get better and better. The treatment of prostate cancer has advanced, and there is good news for most patients.

Chapter XII

Bladder Cancer

"The greater the ignorance; the greater the dogmatism."
– SIR WILLIAM OSLER (1900)

The topic of bladder cancer also deserves an entire book. As this book is a simple manual meant for patients and primary care physicians, I'll be brief.

Doctors suspect bladder cancer when we see blood in the urine. In women, we must be sure the blood is not contamination from menstrual flow. Guidelines for *how much blood in the urine is abnormal* change with every review. Lately, "too much" has been determined to be more than four red blood cells per high power field when viewed under a light microscope. If a patient has this degree of hematuria (blood in the urine), they should be referred to a urologist. Truth be told, however, MOST people with blood in their urine do not have bladder cancer.

One day one of my favorite gynecologists called on my cell phone. She said, "I've just found a solid bladder mass in a 19-year-old college soccer player. She is the picture of health and I was doing a pelvic ultrasound because she has no menses."

I was on the verge of scoffing because I'd never seen bladder cancer in a person so young. Then I remembered gynecologists are very good with ultrasound because they scan pregnant uteri, and this particular doctor is very smart and never an alarmist. She went on to say, "The girl's mom was in the room and saw the mass and is freaked out. Could you please see her today?" My schedule was packed, but like always, I said, *sure*...thinking to myself that *this is likely an unnecessary procedure.*

The patient underwent cystoscopy (examining the bladder with a scope) while her mother watched. Up until the moment I could see inside her bladder, I felt guilty for subjecting this healthy young woman to an uncomfortable and probably needless procedure.

And then, the four of us (me, my nurse, the patient, and her mother) gasped at once. A ten-centimeter (about four inches) cancer was obvious to all. The patient stayed calm while the mother became hysterical. I never again questioned my gynecology colleagues about their ultrasound findings.

This case illustrates how cunning and surprising bladder cancer can be. The patient's only symptom was mild urinary frequency, and her gynecologist found six red blood cells per field in her urine, which is barely above normal. In my career, 95% of patients with blood in their urine did not have cancer, but the other five percent did. Because of our diligence and abundance of caution, this young woman was cured.

TYPES OF BLADDER CANCER:
- Transitional Cell Cancer (TCC) or Urothelial Bladder Cancer (90-95%)
- Squamous Cell Cancer (rare)
- Adenocarcinoma (rare)
- Sarcoma (very rare)

CAUSES OF BLADDER CANCER:

- Cancer starts when cells undergo mutation or changes in the genes and DNA.
- THE NUMBER ONE CAUSE OF BLADDER, URETER AND RENAL PELVIS TUMORS IS CONTACT WITH TOBACCO PRODUCTS! Smoking, extensive second-hand smoke, pipes, and cigars are all proven to contribute.
- DNA mutation is more common with aging.
- Males have bladder cancer more commonly than females.
- Exposure to chemicals (arsenic, dyes, rubber, leather and textile manufacturing, paint products) is a risk factor.
- Chronic infection and inflammation of the bladder (in some countries the parasitic disease schistosomiasis) contribute.
- Family history of bladder cancer or Lynch syndrome (hereditary nonpolyposis colorectal cancer-HNPCC) is a factor and people with this syndrome in their family should consider screening.

PREVENTION:

- Don't smoke or spend much time around people who do!
- Avoid strong industrial chemicals.
- Eat a variety of brightly colored fruits and vegetables to increase antioxidants and decrease free radicals which can damage DNA and contribute to mutations. Research in diet and its effect on our biology is ongoing and the details evolve weekly.

DIAGNOSIS:

- Urinalysis involving microscopy

- Specialized urine testing (cytology or urine FISH tests)
- Pelvic and rectal examination
- Cystoscopy with possible bladder biopsy
- CAT scan of the abdomen, pelvis, and sometimes the chest
- Sometimes an MRI
- Sometimes a positron emission tomography (PET) scanning
- Tumor resection for pathology analysis

The most interesting fact about bladder cancer is that the most common type, transitional cell cancer (TCC), can act like two different cancers. Most bladder cancers are low grade and low stage, and are unlikely to cause death. The ones that are not likely to metastasize are those that come back repeatedly. They usually require the doctor to look in your bladder every three to six months for years to remove any new tumors.

I think of them as being similar to basal cell cancer of the skin. Most of these tumors won't kill you, but they are aggravating to manage because they require multiple visits to the doctors and repetitive minor procedures. The worst types of bladder cancer are not common but deadly. They usually require surgery and chemotherapy, although some are amenable to treatment with agents that are placed in the bladder.

The types of cells that line the bladder also line the ureters and the inside of the kidneys. Your urologist will order cystoscopy and CAT scans of these areas to be sure there are no cancers in more than one location. However, 30% of small bladder tumors can be invisible on CAT scan. Even if your scan is normal, you still need the cystoscopy procedure. Ultrasound is not sensitive enough for small tumors and MRI has, in the past, not been cost effective.

The evaluation and treatment of bladder cancer is under constant scrutiny by urologists, oncologists, and radiologists. Each specialty seeks to find earlier diagnosis and less invasive treatment. Bladder cancer care is fairly standardized and researchers from all over the world collaborate to improve that care.

MOST bladder cancer is curable through early detection and careful follow up. If you have blood in your urine, do not ignore it. Please see a urologist.

Chapter XIII

Be Your Own
Health Care Manager

"The great secret of medicine, known to doctors
but still hidden from the public, is that most things
get better by themselves."

– LEWIS THOMAS, M.D.

"If you judge people, you have no time to love them."

–MOTHER TERESA

In 2009 I weighed 217 pounds and was five feet eight inches tall. I had high blood pressure, abnormal blood sugar and triglycerides, and I was on medication for three self-inflicted diseases. At just 52 years old, I was short of breath and had trouble pulling my legs out of the car to stand. My entire day was spent caring for my patients and my family. I had nothing left for me.

Three pivotal events happened in one month. A college-aged male patient posted a review on the internet about me. In the review he said, "She seems nice enough. She has many diplomas on the wall. But, I have trouble taking health advice from a fat doctor. Who wants a fat doctor? If her advice is all that good, why doesn't she take her own advice?" I was furious. How dare he?

One week later, I saw my personal physician, whom I love. He kindly suggested, "Martha, darling, you must start taking care of yourself. If you don't, there won't be enough pills in America to keep you going." For an hour, I hated his guts! I drove straight to my favorite bakery, bought six petit-fours, and gobbled them in the parking lot while I cried.

After the sugar high subsided, I was no longer angry at my doctor or the review, but at myself. I realized I was doing everything for everyone else and if I dropped dead, folks would step over my fat butt and keep going. What was I doing? I was treating my body like a waste dump and it was beginning to resemble one.

While I drove home sobbing, I thought about who could help me dig out of this mess I'd made of my health. I remembered my friend Dr. Frenesa Hall and sat in my driveway and called her, still crying and shaking and wiping snot from my face.

I knew I had to change. She kindly and calmly talked me through the idea of a year-long program to help me re-establish good habits. After she steered me to a food coach, I recorded everything I ate and called him every week to discuss my successes and my failures. This held me accountable.

I started a mild exercise routine and progressed slowly. At my age, one major goal was to not get hurt. I couldn't do the exercises I used to do, when I was able to swim two miles and roller blade 20 miles, but I could do something. I couldn't think about the past; I had to move steadily forward from where I was now. Dr. Hall stressed that it was important to not be rigid about anything.

I used my mind to envision better health. I didn't focus on the scales even though I did weigh once a week and record it for the coach. I knew a person's weight fluctuated by one or two pounds depending on hydration status and sodium intake. I used hypnotherapy to help deal with the strong emotions driving my overeating, and began to see my health as the starting point for my entire life. I realized that if I did not have my own health, I was good for nobody.

Some days I was driven by spite. I hated that guy who wrote about the fat doctor, but he spurred me on. This impertinent little Googler was right. Who wants to take health advice from an unhealthy person? I started to feel better and was rewarded with better moods and better sleep. My feet, knees, and hips didn't like the exercise at first but eventually everything worked better. My chronic constipation improved. My terrible 3:00 p.m. sugar cravings stopped.

By the time I lost 20 pounds, I was off pills for high blood pressure, diabetes, and high cholesterol. Over two years, I lost 43 pounds and my metabolism normalized.

I wish I could report perfection, but that's not the truth. Over the last ten years, I have gained and lost the same ten pounds. I view it as a form of insanity. I do everything correctly for four months and feel great. Then somebody has a birthday and I eat sugary desserts and the cycle starts over.

I no longer go to the bakery. In fact, I can't remember the name of the baker. I don't miss lying and telling her, "I'm having another party." I definitely don't gobble petit fours in the bakery parking lot. However, I do fall off the wagon a bit. I need five days of exercise per week. I need no more than 2000 calories per day of quality food to feel great. All my calories need to contain nutrients.

Some weeks I just can't do it. Anything that interrupts my sleep cycle is a trigger. If I get too tired, I crave sugar. Sugar and wheat make my muscles and joints feel inflamed and I don't want to exercise. When I don't exercise, I can't sleep well. No exercise and no sleep and my colon won't work well. And I spiral down. Then I again recall those hurtful words. "Nobody wants a fat doctor," and "If you don't take care of yourself, there won't be enough pills in America to save you," and I start over.

I don't manage food perfectly. But I see it as medicine. With fewer medications and doctor's visits, I'm able to spend that time and money on fun vacations. I have accomplished these goals through lifestyle changes. I made these changes while working an 80-hour work week. If I could do it, you can do it too.

FOOD

Patients frequently ask me, "What should I eat?"

After years of traveling, I am convinced that Americans are the most diet-obsessed people in the world. As a culture, we're looking for the holy grail of food. I've seen many diet fads come and go while our population became more and more obese. It is frightening to see the ever-increasing rate of childhood obesity.

One visit to a big box store will show anyone our basic problem. Carts are piled high with processed foods full of carbohydrates and sugar. When I stand in line at the grocery, I see families with ten frozen pizzas, frozen chicken nuggets, premade foods of every type, sugary cereals, and cookies and doughnuts. I see high-fat ground hamburger. I see parents struggling to get their kids to sports activities and throw something at them to eat on the way to the next activity. Many families are too busy to cook good food at home, which is expensive, time consuming, and not their priority.

Our grocery cart is now filled with fruits, vegetables, quality proteins, nothing processed, and little sugar. We attempt to keep the white foods – bread, rice, pasta and potatoes – to a minimum. On a good week, we have one dessert per week. We have instituted "cheat day" at the suggestion of my former food coach. We try to eat very well six days a week and for one day eat anything we want, in small portions.

I am NO dietician. But from many years of observing patients, myself, friends, and people in general, I believe different people need different diets. I am absolutely certain there is no one perfect diet for everyone. A muscled, six-foot-five 240-pound man will certainly need more protein to power his frame than a five-foot wisp of a woman. Common sense is our best guide. I'm also impressed that most people do know what to eat, but for many reasons choose not to follow their own wisdom. It is rare to find a person who truly does not know what to eat.

I have seen great success with the DASH diet, which was developed by the NIH 30 years ago to help lower blood pressure without medication. Supposedly the combination of nutrients in the diet symbiotically works together for maximum health. Most adults are healthier on the DASH diet. There are books written about it. It was voted the "best diet" by dieticians worldwide. I have used it for years in kidney stone formers.

MY EXPERIENCE HAS SHOWN THAT MOST PATIENTS SHOULD:
- Eat little to no processed food. If you cannot pronounce it, do not eat it!
- If it comes in a box or bag, eat little of it.
- Eat organic fresh foods whenever available.
- Avoid sugar, particularly sugary beverages.
- Completely avoid trans-fatty acids. Hydrogenated oils are produced by adding hydrogen to vegetable oil to increase shelf life of foods. These chemicals change your blood fats and increase plaque formation in arteries. Everyone agrees

hydrogenated oils should be eliminated from the diet. How could anything that keeps food fresh for a year be healthy?

- Eat a varied diet. Micronutrients are contained in all kinds of foods.
- Make sure you have enough protein for your body and your activity level. For most women, 50–60 grams per 24 hours and for most men 60–80 grams per 24 hours works. If you choose one of the many KETO diets, you might make kidney stones.
- For me, I had to realize that if I bought it, I would eat it. I plan our food for the week, make a list of exactly what we're going to eat, and my husband does the shopping. He is good at avoiding contraband.
- Fiber supplements help normalize my blood sugar, decrease my food cravings, and help me eat smaller portions. I worked with a company called Unicity and took a product called Balance. My husband was not willing to do anything costly and so he used psyllium and ate an apple at lunch most days. Both filled us up and curbed our appetites.
- When my schedule was crazy, I did a lot of food prep on Sunday afternoon and froze much of our food to make meals easy during the work week.

SLEEP

How does sleep help you lose weight and be healthier?

Again, I'm no sleep expert. But I observed that many patients treated for sleep apnea lost weight. The improved sleep also decreased the number of times they got up at night to urinate and their urinary frequency, urgency, and urge incontinence improved or disappeared. Chronic stress and poor sleep lead to increased cortisol levels. Increased cortisol raises blood sugar and blood pressure and can lead to diabetes, hypertension, heart attack, and stroke. Depression, low libido, poor memory, increased chance of accidents, and poor immunity also occur with poor sleep. Good sleep lowers risks.

To find out how much sleep you need, look at the National Sleep Foundation site.

If your partner notices you stop breathing at times during the night, or that you snore or snort loudly, please tell your primary care doctor and consider seeing a sleep specialist. Many of my patients reported their snoring went away after they achieved normal body weight.

I have never been a good sleeper. As a child, I had night terrors and walked in my sleep. When I became a surgeon and took trauma call, my sleep patterns worsened. Over many years of getting calls all night, I developed great anxiety about sleep. An hour before bedtime, I'd start to worry about getting called by the hospital and not being able to go back to sleep.

After 30 years of sleep interruption, I realized I had to do something. I found a good hypnotherapist who routinely treated sleep disturbances and worked with her. I'm still not a great sleeper. But five nights a week, I get at least seven hours of sleep and my health is much better for it. Good sleep also cured my grumpiness and afternoon sugar cravings.

EXERCISE

First of all, I must disclose that I hate exercise. I am very cerebral and not athletic. I have tried every exercise and the only ones I enjoy are ballroom dancing and swimming, both of which are quite inconvenient. However, the body is designed to move and needs exercise to be healthy.

I get out of bed and complain a lot on my way to my basement. I invested in a treadmill, exercise bike, yoga mat, tap dancing floor, free weight bench, rack of weights, rowing machine, and elliptical. The exercise room is my least favorite place on earth, but it's cheaper than going to the doctor, undergoing lots of expensive tests, and taking costly life-long medications. I exercise because I don't want to be a fat old lady with a bag full of pills. I listen to music for motivation and watch educational videos from *The Teaching Company.* Their courses run 30 minutes and that's the amount of cardio I routinely do.

My husband and I swim one or two days per week, which I enjoy, but swimming may be too time consuming for someone working a full-time job. Swimming and sitting in the hot tub afterwards is our treat.

The body cannot be healthy without exercise. For most people who have not exercised their entire lives, getting started is a daunting task. My best medical advice is to go slow. Keep your expectations low. If you are over 50, your muscles might be stronger than your tendons. Many people decide to get healthier and instead end up in the office of the orthopedic surgeon, either because they hired a trainer who does not know how to help older people, or they tried to perform as they did in their 30s.

Again: Start slow! Walk from five to 15 minutes per day. If you are more than 30 pounds over your ideal body weight, your feet, ankles, knees, hips and back will thank you for slow steady progression. If you are five feet tall, your bones and joints were designed to carry less than 110 pounds.

Do not do very strenuous exercise until you get close to your normal weight. If you try to run with 50 extra pounds on your frame, your body will quickly let you know you've made a mistake. Once your legs are stronger from walking, take the stairs.

Again, make slow progress. Do one flight for a month, then move up to two.

Patience is needed. You need to realize that you did not get unhealthy in one year. You will not get healthy in a few weeks. My own one-year plan turned into a two-year plan. For me, the trouble was food.

I was eating the same portions as my husband, who has twice the muscle mass. According to the physiology experts, at rest, doing nothing, muscle burns more calories than fat. So doing our favorite thing, sitting on the couch reading, he was burning more fuel than me. Over time, I realized I needed 30% less food than him. Boy, was I resentful! When I put together our afternoon snack of an apple and dark chocolate, he got 2/3 of the apple and two chocolate squares. I got 1/3 of the apple and a single square. His snack was not served with love. It came with a hefty dose of jealousy…until my weight started to come off.

Motivation is key. I have never been a particularly vain woman. During my years of surgical training and schooling, I wore no makeup, a constant pony tail, scrubs, and glasses. For years, I may not have even looked in the mirror before going out the door in the morning. Also, I hate to shop. So looking good in my clothes and being a smaller size were never adequate motivation. My motivation was to stay well and not become acquainted with every doctor in town. I did not want to feel poorly on a daily basis. I did not want to spend my hard-earned money having tests and paying for pills. I wanted to use my money to travel and enjoy time with my husband and to run, jump, and play as I aged.

Everyone has to find their own motivation. Maybe it's to be healthy enough to enjoy your grandkids. Maybe it's to play golf until you are 90. Maybe your motivation is to honor the temple of your body that God gave to you as a birthright. Maybe you are fed up with doing things for others and you've decided to take care of you. I don't know what motivates others. But if you can find motivation within yourself and apply patience through discipline and perseverance, you will become healthier. You will spiral up the same way you spiraled down.

My life's work has been studying human behavior. In order to be someone's doctor, you have to figure out who they are and what makes them tick. Before I was a medical doctor, I planned to be a wildlife biologist. I went so far as to do an internship in Washington, DC at the Interior Department's U.S. Fish and Wildlife Service.

I studied endangered species. For 45 years, I have read basic science research, and not only the required medicine and urology. I read about bats and marine life and physics and chemistry and sea turtles. After all these years of reading the science of creatures, I am absolutely certain of one thing: Humans are the only group trying to kill themselves with their habits every day. Wolves do not become sedentary and fat. Bats do not eat foods that make them feel bad, make them sick, and cause them to go on dialysis. All other beings seem to have a "governor" telling them to eat, drink, move around, and follow the cycles of nature. Only man seeks to destroy himself with bad habits.

We are the only ones gambling and shopping away our financial security, having sex in risky scenarios, eating to the point of killing ourselves, imbibing alcohol and drugs to extreme, smoking, gaming, staring at the idiot box every night, texting while driving, assaulting our bodies with repetitive plastic surgeries, and taking bags full of prescription drugs instead of riding our exercise bike. We are unique. There may be a few neurotic pets living with neurotic humans, but most animals are not slowly committing suicide.

If you are sensitive, stop reading right here because you're not going to like my next opinion.

I am no fan of our current health care system. Much could be improved. But every time I hear the news reporting negative things about the outcomes of our system, I want to scream and shout and thrash about.

The truth is that many Americans are daily trying to ruin their lives with stupid habits. We are causing 80% of our own diseases. The pharmaceutical industry, the hospitals, the doctors, the nurses, and our very expensive technology are helping us to live longer and longer even though we fight them every day! That is the big picture truth of American health. These entities the media loves to demonize are keeping us alive longer and longer despite our habits.

If we want to cut our health care spending and put our money on our enjoyment, it is simple for most people…improve your habits. With a little more movement and a little less pizza over 30 years, you can spend less money at the doctor. Of course there are people who do things as best they can and are either born with a hideous disease or are unlucky and develop such a disease. I feel great compassion for those people. I've had close friends, family members, and wonderful patients who do all they can and still suffer.

Please ponder this statement: "There may be more folks fighting cancer as experts than there are people who have cancer." What an industry "fighting cancer" has become in our culture.

Think of the money we spend on awful "cures" giving people two to four months of extended life. What we know is that most forms of cancer are more difficult to treat and likely to occur and recur in unhealthy people. Brightly colored fruits and vegetables and low-level regular exercise decrease the free radicals associated with cancer. Why not do those simple things? Instead of a long list of why you can't do them, every day make a list of what you could do in those 24 hours to decrease your chance of getting cancer. MOVE AROUND! EAT LESS! It's not magic.

I'm sorry for preaching and being self-righteous. I got fat. I was on a bunch of pills. I got to know lots of nice and well-intentioned doctors. They helped me. I quit trying to daily commit suicide with the wrong food and no exercise. Please be smarter than me!

The final truth is exactly what my doctor told me, "If you don't give your body the basic ingredients of health in the form of sleep, exercise, and food, there will not be enough pills and procedures in America to save you from yourself."

Chapter XIV

Meditation and Mind Management

"Whatever an enemy might do to an enemy, or a foe to a foe, the ill-directed mind can do to you even worse."

– SIDDHARTHA GAUTAMA (BUDDHA)

"There is nothing either good or bad, but thinking makes it so…"

– SHAKESPEARE'S HAMLET

"You become what you think about all day long."

– EARL NIGHTINGALE FROM "THE STRANGEST SECRET"

For my entire career I watched patients handle disease and life with many belief systems. I observed them use a cancer diagnosis to completely change their lives and get the lives they wanted.

I've watched other patients get the same diagnosis, fall into despair, and die angry and miserable. To this day, I don't understand why people react the way they do or how we make the choices we make. Out of fear and sheer need, patients and their loved ones shared their most intimate secrets with me. I sought every day to understand human nature and yet it is more mysterious now than when I began seeking.

Despite my ignorance about people's choices, I have noticed repetitive patterns. One that fascinates me is *what a person chooses to think creates their personal experience.* This statement does not apply to fleeting thoughts. It applies to the daily ideas we massage and repeat to ourselves. It's the background music of our lives. It's the underlying theme to all we do and all we believe. It's frequently what motivates us.

There are three books and one pamphlet that have influenced me to change my own habits of thinking. In 1995 I stumbled upon the book *The Science of Mind* by Ernest Holmes. It is a 750-page tome that I read during a time of seeking answers through self-help books. It contains some of what scientists might consider "psychobabble." But it helped me to realize my thinking was causing my chronic dissatisfaction.

I began to see my life as a four-legged stool. I began to actively seek a meaningful spiritual life. I realized my thoughts created my emotions. I learned I could manipulate both my emotions and physical body by managing my thoughts. I watched my blood pressure and heart rate rise in response to angry and resentful thoughts. I could make my muscles tense to the point of pain by rehearsing scenarios in which I felt victimized. I noticed that watching the news was not healthy for me.

So I began to control what I read, to whom I spoke, what I said, and finally, my own thoughts. If a person repeatedly caused negative physical responses, I avoided them. I realized that what

I said, what I ate, what I read, what I wrote, and what I thought created me, and those were all choices over which I had control.

Two people can have the same experience, with one being happy and the other not. One day I was traveling from my home in midtown Atlanta to my office near the Perimeter. I drove north on GA-400 and the traffic was very busy as always. As I was singing along with Marvin Gaye and tapping on my steering wheel, I may have made a lane shift that wasn't the best-timed move.

Waiting at the tollbooth while a driver ahead of me had difficulty paying, I gazed into my rearview mirror and saw a man waving his hands in the air and screaming at me. He pointed, shouted, and made "Mr. Meany faces," to express his dissatisfaction with my driving, which was not up to his standards.

I waved, smiled, and continued to listen to Marvin. Instead of calming down, he seemed even more agitated. After we finally made it through the toll line, he sped up to pass me and gave me the finger as he did so. Fifteen minutes later, I walked into an exam room in my office to see my first patient of the day. Guess who?

The man was there for his yearly rectal exam. I stood in the doorway and smiled. His eyes were wide and his breathing shallow and fast as recognition flooded over both of us. He chose to not acknowledge what had happened. On physical examination, his pulse and blood pressure were high. His exam was difficult because his sphincter was in spasm. His body demonstrated his thoughts and his tense muscles were not helpful to our purpose. He and I were in the same situation at the toll booth. Both of us were concerned about being late. I chose to enjoy the time listening to music that fed my soul. He made different choices. We were great examples of *what I choose to think creates my personal experience.* I don't know for sure, but I suspect his visit would have been easier if his muscles had been less tense.

Around 1996 I met Dr. Herbert Benson, the famous author and Harvard cardiologist who wrote *Timeless Healing: The Power and Biology of Belief.* If you can only discipline yourself to read one book about how the mind and its thoughts affect your body, this is the one. Dr. Benson does a marvelous job of explaining in simple terms how thoughts create health and disease. He called to the fore the idea that 75% of all primary care doctor's office visits are stress related. His chapter on the nocebo effect reinforced much of what I learned at Charity Hospital in New Orleans. The nocebo effect is when a patient develops symptoms or side effects of a therapy because they believe the problem will occur. I saw many people whose belief that a hex or voodoo curse had been placed on them was so strong that they developed disease. Unmitigated terror can bring about fatal results.

The opposite of the nocebo response is Dr. Benson's "relaxation response." He showed in a scientific manner how the fear-based fight-or-flight response increased metabolism, blood pressure, heart rate, and muscle tension. He also demonstrated that these body functions are decreased by the relaxation response. He explained that, "Long term and regular elicitation of the relaxation response has enormous benefit to the body."

Through meditation, prayer, use of mantras, guided imagery, breathing exercises, focused walks, yoga, tai chi, music, and sitting in nature, we can induce the relaxation response and heal our bodies. It all starts with calming the mind.

Another book that has been a powerful aid for me is *The Power of NOW* by Eckhart Tolle. There is also some of what I call woo-woo stuff in this book. What I learned is that I am totally responsible for my inner peace. Nobody else is responsible for my happiness. My happiness is not controlled by outside events or circumstances. And my happiness depends on right now.

I can't change the past. I cannot control the future. What I have is the moment in front of me and what I allow myself to think about now. Some of my sickest patients carried horrible burdens from child abuse, sexual and verbal abuse, and infidelity. Those things happened to them. They were real. But rehashing them in their minds day in and day out was ruining their current lives. Learning to accept that the terrible things happened, forgiving everyone involved, and realizing that NOW is not then, helped some to heal and move on to create lives worth living. Others could not make that transition. They lived in the past and carried it with them everywhere.

One beautiful and intelligent fifty-year-old woman told me at every visit of her rape by a neighbor at age twelve. Over a decade the story never changed and her unwillingness to consider therapy never wavered. She held steadfast to her belief that, "He did this to me; it's his entire fault, so why should I go to therapy?" She endured eleven laparoscopies with other doctors trying to cure her pelvic pain. She needed multimodal therapy with psychological counselling and physical therapy being a major part of her treatment.

What I learned from her is that her life was defined by that event. Her neighbor not only stole her innocence, but by her inability to forgive him and move on...she allowed him to steal her life. She never trusted men and spent all of her money and time at well-meaning doctors who never helped her. Her body was sickened by her thoughts. She could not get into the now. No surgery, pill, or test could heal her. Her deep-seated fear kept her from considering treatments that might have helped. She kept returning to me because she trusted me, and I never did anything to make her worse. She sensed that I cared about her. But in the decade she came to me, she was never willing to face her fear and follow the treatment I advised.

My life, like all lives, has had sorrow and pain. None of us lives a completely charmed life. The thing that has helped me to get beyond the experiences that hurt me most has been a 22- page pamphlet by Dr. Emmet Fox entitled *The Seven Days Mental Diet*. Our minds form a constant stream of thoughts, most of which we are not totally aware of having. But thoughts create energy and energy creates movement.

This little jewel of a book gave me specific instructions in learning about thoughts that do not serve me and how to change them. For over 15 years, I have done exactly what the pamphlet suggests. Every January, I go on a mental diet where I observe my own thoughts continuously for seven days. It might sound easy and simple, but it is not. It is profound and life changing.

Playing in the background for most of my life was that song… *nobody loves me, everybody hates me…I'm gonna go eat worms.* I had a crazy core belief system, which I have no idea from whence it came, that I had to be as perfect as possible or nobody would like me. My motivation for nearly everything I did was that I had to be better than most to be considered OK.

Because I was adopted, I wondered if my prior life could have had anything to do with my belief system. I was adopted into a nice, average family and can see nothing that happened there to support my beliefs about myself. I could have spent many years in therapy to figure out why I thought as I did, but what I really needed was to CHANGE MY THINKING!

It really did not matter why I played that theme song. It was nuts and had to go. It drove me. It created what I came to call "the bitch with the list." She woke me up every day at four in the morning to exercise and make everyone's gourmet lunch and wash clothes at dawn. She made me into an enormous overachiever. Her voice pushed me and gave me many wonderful things in life. But the thinking and striving nearly ruined my health.

By following exactly what Dr. Fox suggests in the pamphlet, I have changed the thoughts that have not served me well. I have created thoughts that make my life better and better. You can do it too.

ACTION STEPS TO CONSIDER
- Read and follow *The Seven Days Mental Diet* pamphlet.
- Read *Timeless Healing* by Herbert Benson.
- Begin a daily meditation practice.
- Read and reread *The Way to Love* by Anthony De Mello.
- If you have had major life trauma, seek psychological help.
- Know that physical disease can originate in the mind.
- Believe that your physical ailments may require both conventional and nonconventional medicine to achieve your best health.

THE POWER OF MEDITATION

Every day patients asked me "How do I meditate?" Remember I am a surgeon by training and temperament. I am no meditation expert. With that disclaimer, I will tell you that meditation is made too complex by modern "gurus." It's nothing other than sitting quietly and letting your thoughts cease.

When I first started doing it, my mind was like a gerbil on crack. Every time I'd sit down to meditate, my mind would get worse, as thoughts increased and became even darker. The more I tried to calm my mind, the greater the energy it created towards chaos. For me, it was like starting an exercise program: It got worse before it got better.

Start slow and take it easy. Do five minutes in the morning and five minutes in the evening. Sit quietly without interruption and attempt to let your thoughts roll over you. In the beginning, I'd say prayers or mantras and try to take slow deep breaths. One of my favorite mantras is, "God has better ideas than you."

Some days I felt better and some days it almost seemed to make me tenser. But I persevered. Just like exercise…it got better. And just like exercise…some days it still sucks. And, just like exercise, it took six to 12 weeks to become part of my daily routine.

WHAT I GET FROM MY MEDITATION PRACTICE:
- My daily coping skills are better.
- Life doesn't frustrate me as much.
- My sleep is better because I can shut off my mind.
- My creativity has blossomed.
- I'm better able to solve complex problems with less effort.
- My physical health is better.
- I've become more forgiving of myself and others.
- I accept life as it is with less struggle.
- My anxiety is improved.

Resilience is the capacity to recover quickly from difficulties. I think resilience determines whether an individual has a happy life or not. I view resilience as being what I tell myself about what is happening to me. It is at the core of what I choose to believe.

If we live long enough, terrible things happen to all of us. What we believe about these events, the importance we place on them, the stories we tell ourselves about them and the actions we choose to take around them all determine our ability to be happy no matter what. And our ability to be happy no matter what determines the quality of our lives. I have had intermittent success and failure at making myself happy, no matter what, during the course of my 65 years.

On July 4th, 2009, our family was planning a big party. Our invitation stated, *COME FOR GREAT FIREWORKS!* When our guests arrived with casseroles and wine bottles in hand, they were greeted by six firetrucks, eight police cars, a local news helicopter flying over our house, and my children standing in the street crying. An outdoor citronella candle had blown up, set the roof on fire, and burned our home to the ground and everything we owned along with it. By anyone's standards, this was a terrible event.

As the house burned, I was on the phone talking to the emergency room about two of my patients who were passing kidney stones. I stood in the street out of the way of the wonderful firefighters and explained to the ER doctor that I'd have to find another urologist to care for these patients because I could not get out of my subdivision due to the fire trucks. Of course, they thought I was teasing.

The shocked partygoers left, the fire was kept from damaging our neighbors' houses, and my husband and I stood in front of what remained of our home. We had just finished a complete remodel of the kitchen two days before. We hugged, held hands, and eventually laughed at the irony, devastated but grateful that nobody was injured. A woman we did not know well walked up to us and gave us the key to her home and directions on how to get there. She said she'd stay with her boyfriend and we could use her house until we got settled. She was our angel that night.

We had NOTHING left but our cars, which we'd moved to use the space for a bouncy gym we'd rented for the children attending the party. My husband was wearing a swimsuit and I was wearing a sundress, both with cheap plastic flip-flops. We drove to the hospital and stole a few sets of scrubs, went on to Target for basic toiletries and moved into the house of the lady we didn't know. Just like all people in catastrophic scenarios, we did the next right thing until we had a functioning life again.

We never missed a day of work. Seeing people with cancer and other life-threatening situations made us realize we could have it worse. Our gratitude grew by focusing on the fact that our children were not burned. People figured out where we were staying (I've never known how) and food began to appear on the doorstep every night. Folks cleaned out their closets and brought their clothes to us. The kindness was outrageous. However, the biggest part of our getting past this very hard life event was the stories we told ourselves.

We laughed as our kids accused me of burning down the house because I'm a powerful witch who never liked the floor plan. We realized that the vast amount of stuff we'd accumulated was weighing us down. We drew together as a couple. We quickly realized that we could fight over a million little things and end up divorced, or we could figure out who was good at what and work through the process. We learned much about each other that would have taken us years to learn otherwise.

One thing we found was that I am good at conflict resolution. I could deal with the insurance companies, the mortgage people, the rental companies, the lawyers, and the interfaces between all of them. He turned out to be an excellent decorator and was able to envision a house better than the one we had. He upgraded our home in many ways by shopping the market and working with the builder. He picked out everything and I worked to get the money to pay for it.

It was a horrendous process. Many negative and heart-wrenching events happened throughout those two years, but we told ourselves stories of hope and faith and rebuilt better than before. Our bond was tighter as we came to believe there was nothing we could not face together. Our mutual respect, our trust, and out sense of humor all grew. Our children learned that you can lose all your stuff and still have a good life. The only things that we miss and mourn 13 years later are our family photos of people who have died. We had them stored in multiple places, but not on the cloud. We had never envisioned a scenario in which we'd lose all we had.

I tell this to demonstrate the power of resilience and story. The meaning we assign to the events that happen determines our happiness. We told ourselves that we would build back better than ever and believed it. That is resilience in action. We were grateful no lives were lost. We saw that as a huge gift. I won't pretend we did not squabble with each other. It took six months to figure out who was going to do what in this huge long-term project of rebuilding our lives. We developed a skill that has saved us many times, which is to acknowledge that some days suck. In fact, some weeks suck. But, at the end of the day, no matter how aggravated we are at each other, we hug and say, "I love you. Better luck tomorrow." That is our way of acknowledging we aren't happy, but we are committed to being happy.

Another example of how the story we tell ourselves determines our happiness is the story of my adoption.

Adoption is an amazing thing. Unfortunately, many people who are adopted are never happy. They spend their lives feeling abandoned and fantasizing about their "real parents." They take on a victim persona and use their adopted status to create chaos.

I had periods in my life when I struggled with these feelings, until I finally told myself a story that frees me. Both of my biological parents were severe alcoholics. They probably had many wonderful characteristics, but I was the lucky baby to have been adopted into a loving and much more happily functioning family.

I am grateful to have had the parents and wonderful extended family that I have had. I see them as a gift.

I also feel grateful to my biological mother for having me. She could have made other decisions. As an adult, I have been blessed to meet her extended families, who are some of the nicest people I've ever met. They too are a huge gift.

It turns out that my cousin Bettye was 15 years old and at the hospital when I was born. She wondered her entire life *what happened to that baby?* Today we love each other and I'm part of her family. We did not meet until "the baby" was sixty years old.

I was also excited to learn that I'm related to one of my favorite authors, Pat Conroy, by marriage. I happened into the Conroy Center in Beaufort, South Carolina, to see their amazing collection. I was guided by a delightful woman who later came to realize I was the baby her family had given for adoption. Many of them wondered what had happened to me. I was known in their extended family as "The Lucky Baby." She researched me because we had hit if off so well and wrote a letter to tell me that I was related to her husband.

It would be one choice to bemoan my plight and wonder, "what if?" But due to resilience, I am grateful to know these wonderful folks and glad they came into my life. I choose to be entertained by the story and believe that it all happens exactly as it should. What I believe is a choice. My beliefs create emotions and emotions create the tone of my life. The tone of my life creates actions. I choose to see these new family members as gifts and visit them and enjoy them when I can. Life happens for our greatest good. You really can choose happiness.

There is a famous 12-step book that says, "Serenity is inversely proportional to your expectations." My Dad taught me that I was to expect life would not always go as I thought best. If I was lucky enough to own a car, it would break down and need tires and oil from time to time. He suggested I save my money to be prepared for the cracked window, flat tire, and filter changes that were part of the gift of being wealthy enough to have a car. He taught me to expect the unexpected. He taught me that if I became unhappy every time my day did not go as I thought it should, I'd be unhappy much of the time.

Dad believed that most of the misery of the world was caused by folks being upset that they did not get something they wanted or were afraid of losing something they had. He taught me that what I perceive as a problem is simply me not getting what I expected. He taught me that other people's opinions of me are nothing to be concerned about. He told me not to be swayed by others because, "Little girl, you are neither as good nor as bad as they say."

I found his advice very helpful when I read my reviews as a doctor on the internet. Some patients thought I was their savior and some thought I was the devil incarnate. I took both with confidence that I am *neither as good nor as bad as they say.* The less I expect things to be a certain way, the happier I am. A post-it note on my computer says *GOD HAS BETTER IDEAS THAN ME.*

On my best days, I practice resilience by changing my expectations into gratitude. Another important lesson I learned from Dad was that most people are doing the best that they can on any given day. He taught me to *FORGIVE EVERYONE FOR EVERYTHING.* Part of being resilient is to keep my eye on my ball. If I am truly taking care of myself and my responsibilities, I have no energy left to drag around resentments towards other people for not meeting my expectations. This lighter load frees up my energy to focus on doing what I need to do.

I'm still not Jesus or Mother Teresa. I get mad and have to put myself in time-out. I keep a zipper on the dash of the car to remind myself to *zip it up* when my husband drives aggressively. But I have the time and energy to be resilient because I choose not to live in resentment and fear and regret and victimhood.

Chapter XV

Toxins

"Observe due measure; moderation is best in all things."
– GREEK POET HESIOD (700 BC)

TYPES OF TOXINS:
- Chemical
- Biological
- Physical
- Radiation
- Behavioral

I started to omit this chapter because our world has generated a plethora of confusion around this topic. I can't tell you how many women with dyed hair, fake acrylic nails and faces modeled by injections and Botox came to see me looking for a vegan treatment for their UTIs because, "they didn't want toxins in their body." As a doctor, it's my job to judge no one and help everyone to the best of my ability. Sometimes my patience was challenged during this scenario.

Every day I saw patients with bags full of supplements who refused the one prescription drug likely to treat their problem. I saw folks who should be a size 12 starve themselves down to a size two in the name of "health." I saw folks who should weigh 125 pounds but weighed 250 and were certain none of their medical problems were weight related. *"Judge not, that ye be not judged,"* Matthew 7:1-3, was on another note attached to my computer.

I've watched myself do stupid things repetitively. I have put on and taken off the same weight for 20 years. I believe my behavior around food to be a form of insanity. I have *food schizophrenia*. I eat the way I believe to be perfectly for six weeks and then eat dessert every night for a week. I don't know why humans do things we know are bad for us. The best I've been able to do is moderate.

WHAT IS *PROVEN*?
- Air pollution is bad for us.
- Water pollution is bad for us.
- Chemicals in food are bad for us. As I said in an earlier chapter, if you can't pronounce it, DON'T EAT IT. (An example: polycyclic aromatic hydrocarbons = can't pronounce it, don't eat it)
- Diets high in sugar are toxic.
- Fat cells aren't sitting there doing nothing. They produce unhealthy compounds. So get as close to your ideal body weight as possible. Any reduction in fat content is good. When you decrease fat, you decrease the fat cells' factory of toxic chemicals.
- Alcohol, tobacco, drugs (including prescription), and supplements should be avoided if possible. If it's not possible, work with your physician to moderate drug use.

- Toxic relationships cause our bodies to release the same chemicals as are seen in chronic stress. These chemicals, if sustained, are unhealthy.
- Poor sleep in either quantity or quality is toxic. Our bodies must have the rejuvenation found in good sleep.
- Lack of exercise is toxic. We were designed to move.
- I believe chronic FEAR and anxiety cause DIS-EASE.

HOW DOES OUR *BODY* REMOVE TOXINS?

- Exhaling breath
- Sweat
- Urination
- Defecation
- Under some circumstances by vomiting
- Metabolism via the liver and lymphatics and immune system

We must work towards a cleaner environment. Drink clean water, eat healthy food, get a good night's sleep, avoid toxic people, use common sense, know that any pill of any type can be toxic to your body and only take pills you really need under the care of your personal physician, breathe deeply, and move around.

Don't fall for fads. I wish I knew the "best diet." In my over 200,000 interactions with people about what they eat, I am convinced that the proper diet is an individual thing. There is no one diet that works best for most people. But I'm also convinced that if you pay close attention, your body will tell you what to eat.

ALCOHOL

Ten percent of people should never drink alcohol. It is a life-ruining choice for those folks, though I don't know why. Ninety percent can drink in moderation and it may even be healthy in that group. If drinking alcohol sets up a craving such that you want to drink it beyond all reason, you are likely an alcoholic. A beverage that most can imbibe with impunity is deadly in you. Alcoholics Anonymous has been helpful to many.

FOOD ALLERGIES

Some folks have a true allergy to foods like shrimp, green bell peppers, wheat, or peanuts. I don't fully understand food allergies and my allergy immunology buddies don't seem to agree about them either. If you think you might have a gluten allergy, your gastroenterologist can help. If you have systemic reactions to other foods, a board-certified allergist can assist you.

The body is brilliant. If we give it half a chance, it will take excellent care of itself and serve us well for a long time, in most cases.

Chapter XVI

Intuition

"The intellect has little to do on the road to discovery.
There comes a leap in consciousness, call it intuition or
what you will, and the solution comes to you, and you
don't know how or why."

– ALBERT EINSTEIN

One of the most powerful tools available for managing our health is our intuition. Whether you are the doctor or the patient, your intuition is a powerful assistant.

One definition of intuition is the ability to understand something immediately without the need for conscious reasoning. The enemy of intuition is fear. If both the doctor and the patient recognize that most problems can be solved, drop their fear of not being able to solve them, open their minds and hearts to the best option for all without ego or distraction by contempt prior to investigation, intuition can accomplish miracles.

I'm absolutely certain we communicate on levels that are not obvious. Most of us get a hunch that proves to be true. Most of us get a bad feeling about a situation or a person that turns out to be correct. Do not ignore these feelings. Just make sure it's not unfounded fear and if it's not, pay attention and trust your deepest guidance mechanism.

A decade ago a well-known trial lawyer came to see me for his yearly prostate examination. Doctors as a group don't mix well with trial lawyers because we're afraid of medical malpractice suits. American surgeons are among the most "sued" professionals in the world despite being the most educated. I have many lawyers for patients. Long ago, I decided to treat them as I would treat anyone else.

The trial lawyer's urology history, physical examination, and blood work were normal. There was nothing to suggest prostate cancer. But I *knew* he had prostate cancer. Because I am bound by science, I chose not to tell him. That night, I could not sleep. I wrestled with the ethics of telling him what I thought with my intuition versus the scientifically proven data. His referral doctor was one of my best clients and I did not want to expose my intuition to his scrutiny. My conscience got the better of me and I called the lawyer the next day.

I said, "You might think me crazy, but I have to tell you something. I am convinced you have prostate cancer even though all evidence points to your not having it. If you saw ten urologists, nobody would tell you to get a biopsy. Prostate biopsy is uncomfortable and not without possible complications. I want you to know that over the course of my career, when I get strong feelings like I have about you, they have never been wrong."

To my surprise, he said, "I too have intuition. And I feel you have my best interest at heart. Set up the biopsy." We did and he had prostate cancer that was intermediate in grade and stage and he needed therapy. He had a robotic prostatectomy and has had no sign of reoccurrence ten years later.

I wish I could tell you what intuition is. To me, it is God. I never ignore it and advise you don't either.

You are an individual and what works for others may not work for you. Let's say your friend had surgery with a particular doctor and had a great outcome. You see the doctor on your friend's suggestion. At your visit you get an overwhelming feeling that this doctor is not the one for you. Do not ignore that feeling.

Another scenario to consider is that your very trusted and well-liked personal physician suggests a procedure or medicine you have a strong feeling against. Keep looking for other answers. Quality medicine is available in most urban areas. You can get other opinions or see other doctors if the suggested care doesn't sound right for you. Unfortunately, in rural areas, this is not always the case. Many academic centers will see patients with complex problems even if they are not well insured. Seek care at the best academic centers if your local doctors are not experienced in your problem.

In the early days of my surgical training, if I felt a patient would benefit from a procedure, I saw it as my duty to talk them into having that operation. I thought that was part of my job. Over the years, I realized that my job was to give my patients the best information I had available and help them find competent doctors if they chose to explore other options. It was my job to not take my patients' choices as a personal affront when their choices differed from my expert opinion.

In the past few years, we have realized that low grade, low stage prostate cancer does not need aggressive treatment in many men. They can live with it if they have very careful follow-ups. Fifteen years ago, I diagnosed several men with prostate cancer who refused any treatment. I lost sleep and worried and all but begged them to have surgery. I read the current literature on the topic and could not accept their decisions. If my job was not to cure cancer, then what was it?

Every man returned years later, still alive and thriving. They knew something I didn't. If those same men walked in today, I'd happily offer the path they chose despite my insistence. What is this knowing? Is it God? Is it race consciousness? Is it some type of psychic event? I do not know. I just learned to trust it.

If I had a strong feeling that someone was not going to do well with a procedure, I'd ask them to get another opinion. If someone told me they did not want to do something and I thought they had good reasons and were not just acting out of fear, I let it go. I'd suggest you try to not be unduly affected by what you see on the internet. Use it as a tool to help devise questions for your doctor. But please do not believe everything you read, even if it comes from a very sophisticated website. I'd suggest the same for reviews of doctors and hospitals. People get angry and say things that are exaggerated. Don't let that keep you from using services that could benefit you greatly.

Your primary care doctor knows the best doctors and hospitals. They are the ones who hear the complaints and the last thing they want is to have you return with complaints. Ask nurses; they will tell you the truth. Know that sometimes the person with the best skill does not have the best personality. You don't want a really nice guy who is not terribly smart or skilled doing your heart surgery. The best outcome could be with a surgeon whose interpersonal skills are mediocre.

IN SUMMARY:
- Educate yourself before you visit the doctor.
- Prepare your questions and take them to the visit.

- Review the doctor's suggestions and if they seem reasonable, follow them.
- If either the doctor or their advice doesn't feel right, get another opinion.
- Avoid trusting the internet too much.
- Watch out for your own fear.
- Take reviews lightly because many happy customers don't write them.
- Remember that for some things you need an excellent technician and not a charming personality.
- For believers like me, pray about it. Pray before the visit. Pray for your doctor. Know that something bigger than you and bigger than your doctor is guiding the path. If you can't believe in God, believe in Good Orderly Direction and try it anyway.
- The more you use your intuition, the more powerful it becomes.

Chapter XVII

The Future Is Bright

"Identify your problems, but give your power and energy to solutions."

– TONY ROBBINS

I was in the third edit of this book when Mr. Tony Robbins, Dr. Peter Diamandis, and Dr. Robert Hariri published their book *Life Force* (2022). It drove me to read Ray Kurzweil's book *The Singularity is Near: When Humans Transcend Biology* (2005).

Reading these books reminded me of the many changes I've seen in urology. I was drawn to urology initially because I loved open kidney stone surgery. It was dramatic and difficult and technically challenging and the patient received great benefit. Unbeknownst to me, while I dedicated 100 hours a week of my youth to learning that procedure and others, a group of German engineers were perfecting extracorporeal shock wave lithotripsy or ESWL. They made my training obsolete before I finished perfecting my skills! I never did the procedure that drew me into urology after 1990. In ten short years, ESWL took over as the procedure of treatment for many renal stones.

In his book, Robbins points out that information technology, knowledge growth, and innovation are happening faster and faster. With the spread of the internet, improved communication, information sharing, artificial intelligence, and the ability to manipulate our DNA, much is happening to improve our health and longevity.

His chapters on regenerative medicine are excellent. He has long been a leader in rallying people to see how their mindset creates their lives. Now he's gathered teams of experts to help explain the personalized medicine revolution of the future.

If you want to understand some of the DNA advances and you are not a science person, I suggest *Life Force.* I also strongly suggest Walter Isaacson's book *The Code Breaker.*

We have only touched the surface of what can be and is being done with stem cells and DNA gene editing. I believe the future of the human race will be determined by how we use artificial intelligence and allow our DNA to be rearranged. If you want to be left behind, as I was with the open kidney stone surgery, ignore what's coming. But it's coming whether you see it or not, and quickly. I suggest you read trusted sources and learn as much as possible about all the amazing developments. You or someone you love could be offered suboptimal medical care. If you educate yourself about technology, you will be a smarter consumer.

If you had seen me as your urologist in 1988, I might have offered to cut you open from side to side to remove your stone and keep you in the hospital for a week and out of work for a month. I was a smart, diligent, and concerned surgeon. I had "state of the art training." But I was working 100 hours a week just to learn what I needed to care for my patients' immediate concerns. Meanwhile, folks in another part of the world were figuring out how to break up your stone under sedation, keep you in the hospital overnight, and get you back to work in a couple of days.

Knowledge is growing exponentially. Moore's Law is a historical observation that "the number of transistors on a microchip doubles every two years while the cost halves." In extremely simple terms, this is the history of technology. Your phone keeps getting smaller and less expensive but can do more. At the intersection of quantum computing, block chain, robotics, 3-D printing, nanotechnology, artificial intelligence, internet of things (IoT), and the potential of global supply chains lies the future of health care.

I'll give a concrete example of why I think the future is bright and our current system of health care is quickly on the way to being archaic. The structure of DNA was discovered in 1953. It took 13 years and $3 billion to sequence the human genome, which was mostly complete by 2003. By 2005, it took five days and $2,000 to get your genome sequenced. In 2022, it takes eight hours and costs $400.

Science and medicine are progressing faster and faster as our ability to store, compute and communicate information becomes quicker and less expensive. The day is coming when AI produces personalized drugs quickly and affordably.

Trust your doctor, but know you are the one responsible for being a good consumer of health care. There are options for diagnosis and treatment about which even a diligent doctor may not be aware.

PAY ATTENTION AND EDUCATE YOURSELF ABOUT:
- Gene therapy
- CRISPR technologies
- Stem cell technologies
- Food Science

I again encourage you to read *Life Force* to learn more about regenerative medicine and longevity research. Pay particular attention to pages 541-568 to learn about our bright and exciting future in health care. I have no relationship with Robbins and have never even met him. But even as a doctor, I learned from his book and wanted you to have it in your toolkit.

Many of the greatest innovations come from people who are able to look at the big picture and envision solutions. Be the one to look at your health and envision longevity and your best health ever.

I'm complete now. I've told you everything I never had time to tell you in a fifteen-minute office visit. This is my love letter to my patients and to all the primary care people who entrusted me with the care of their precious patients.

Always remember:

"If you would be a real seeker of truth, it is necessary that at least once in your life you doubt, as far as possible, all things."
–RENE DESCARTES

ACKNOWLEDGMENTS

I'd like to thank the Atlanta Writers Club and Mr. George Weinstein for supporting my transition from surgeon to author. Our club is one of the best in the country.

I'd like to thank Mr. David Hancock for trusting me to deliver both fiction and non-fiction. He has many great authors from which to choose and I'm happy to be one of the Morgan James authors. I heard so many negative things about publishers from other authors. I must say that everyone at Morgan James has been enjoyable.

I'd like to thank Mr. Terry Whalin for his guidance and his book *Book Proposals That Sell.* I learned through my medical education to always ask for help from experts. The book proposal process was daunting, but Terry's guidance and his book made the process enjoyable.

I'd like to thank my editor for this project, Mr. David Swan. He did an amazing job and I recommend him highly.

I'm grateful to my beta readers for this project: Warren Hébert, DNP, RN, FAAN is an excellent academic writer and added much professionalism to the book. Richard D. Keegan, DNP, MSN, FNP, BSN, RN provided valuable insight from a nursing standpoint. Richard Barlow, M.D. has been a trusted colleague for many years and was helpful with his suggestions and discernment.

I'm grateful to the Women in Publishing Summit, which was an online writers' conference. In the middle of the pandemic when I had no support for my writing, Alexa Bigwarfe and her team conducted an amazing online writers' conference with speakers from all over the world. That conference enthused me at a time when I was ready to throw two books in the trash.

I'm forever grateful to the many medical professionals who made my career in something I loved possible. Medicine takes a team and I have always enjoyed the best of teams.

My deepest thanks are to my patients. Thank-you for trusting me with your very being. That trust was never taken lightly. Even if I was grumpy and sleepless and at times scared, your best care was always what motivated me.

I'm forever grateful for my education. Kingstree Senior High, The College of Charleston, The Medical University of South Carolina, Tulane Surgery and Tulane Urology, the University of California-Davis and the ongoing education offered by the American Urologic Association contributed to my career. These schools enrolled women in science and medicine at a time when not everyone did. My opinions in this book do NOT necessarily reflect the opinions of these institutions, but I would have had no career without them.

As always, nothing much happens without the help of my husband. Jesse is everything to me. He's a quiet, competent, smart, and giving man. He has made me better than I would otherwise be. His love and support has healed me so I had the wherewithal to help heal others.

ABOUT THE AUTHOR

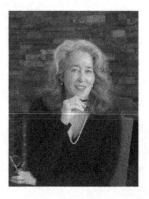

Dr. Martha Boone is one of the first one hundred women board certified in urology. After 23 years of education, she practiced academic urology for five years and private practice for twenty four. She was named TOP DOC in urology in Atlanta for over a decade. Her first novel *The Big Free* fictionalizes her six years at Charity Hospital in New Orleans. Dr. Boone retired to write full-time and travel with her husband.

A free ebook edition is available with the purchase of this book.

To claim your free ebook edition:

1. Visit MorganJamesBOGO.com
2. Sign your name CLEARLY in the space
3. Complete the form and submit a photo of the entire copyright page
4. You or your friend can download the ebook to your preferred device

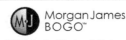

A **FREE** ebook edition is available for you
or a friend with the purchase of this print book.

CLEARLY SIGN YOUR NAME ABOVE

Instructions to claim your free ebook edition:
1. Visit MorganJamesBOGO.com
2. Sign your name CLEARLY in the space above
3. Complete the form and submit a photo of this entire page
4. You or your friend can download the ebook to your preferred device

Print & Digital Together Forever.

Snap a photo

Free ebook

Read anywhere

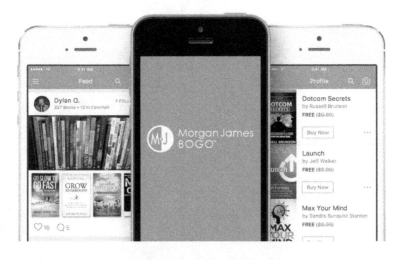